Bowel Nosodes in Homeopathic Practice

Saltire Books   *Saltire Books Limited, Glasgow, Scotland*

Bowel Nosodes in Homeopathic Practice

Third Edition

JOHN SAXTON
BVetMed, VetFFHom, CertIAVH, MRCVS

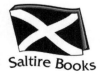
Saltire Books   *Saltire Books Limited, Glasgow, Scotland*

Published by Saltire Books Ltd

18–20 Main Street, Busby, Glasgow G76 8DU, Scotland
books@saltirebooks.com   www.saltirebooks.com

 is a registered trademark

First edition published in 2008
Second edition published in 2012
Reprinted 2016
Third edition published in 2020

Typeset by Type Study, Scarborough, UK in 9¼ on 13½ Stone Serif
Printed and bound in the UK by TJ International Ltd, Padstow, Cornwall

ISBN 978-1-908127-18-1

For Saltire
Project Development: Lee Kayne
Editorial: Steven Kayne
Designer: Phil Barker
Indexer: Laurence Errington

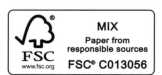

CONTENTS

PREFACE TO THE FIRST EDITION

The general link of the bowel flora to health is now widely recognised and in many cases this finds expression in the widespread use of diets, prebiotics and probiotics. Helpful as these approaches may be, their use is essentially one that applies external solutions to the internal problems of health. In contrast the bowel nosodes, produced from bacterial agents associated with healthy curative reactions in the body, affect the bowel flora by initiating permanent changes in the internal dynamic of the body, thus acting on the disease state from a deeper level. For this reason they are more than just a group of remedies linked together by a similar source – they present unique opportunities for the treatment of chronic disease and their nature and uses are distinct. They have connections at the deepest levels with other remedies, and because of this can be used to stimulate, expand and augment the actions of those remedies. Compared to the total number of remedies available to the practitioner, the bowel nosodes form a small and often overlooked group, underrepresented in many materia medicas and general repertories.

The origins and development of the bowel nosodes lie in the field of human medicine and their importance and usefulness is out of all proportion to their numbers. Their applications encompass both the human and veterinary fields, as indicated by the near parity between the numbers of human and animal cases that are presented in this book. These cases have been selected to demonstrate the basic guidelines governing the use of the bowel nosodes, which are applicable to all species. Chronic disease is the area that is of major clinical importance in the modern age. There is a resonance between the bowel nosodes and the miasms, and the nosodes provide one means of addressing the miasmatic influences that are so active in chronic illness. Yet on occasion the bowel nosodes find employment also in the more acute situation. Nevertheless, many otherwise experienced homeopaths appear to shy away from this group of remedies without fully exploring their potential.

One reason for this may be that although there are already other texts on the bowel nosodes, these tend to concentrate on their materia medica. In general the philosophy behind the group, their development and clinical indications are discussed only superficially. Thus the concept behind them appears often to remain obscure. These other works have their place, but without an understanding of the rationale behind the bowel nosodes the best use will not be made of them in the clinical situation. Thus it was clear that there was a need for a new point of reference, one that drew together all the isolated pieces of information and placed them within both an historical and developmental context plus that of current homeopathic thought and practice. The development of the bowel nosodes is traced as a means of understanding their position and true role in the healing process, and the materia medica of each is discussed, with appropriate case histories.

A knowledge of the basic principles of homeopathy is assumed and all references to the *Organon* apply to the 6th edition, edited by Wenda Brewster O'Reilly. Also, different spellings of 'homeopathy' will be found in the book: in the text the more modern format is used whereas where references are quoted the format found in the original is retained.

It is hoped that this work will be of interest and use to all practitioners and students of homeopathy, encouraging the more widespread use of a group of remedies that are still undervalued by many, whilst at the same time increasing their usefulness to those who are already aware of their potential.

PREFACE TO THE SECOND EDITION

The opportunity of a new edition has been taken to review the whole text, and although there have been no major changes to most of the previous chapters, all have had some additions. Chapters 1 and 2 have been expanded to provide fuller discussion of various aspects of the context and background to the subjects that were mentioned only briefly before, notably the relationship to and contrast with probiotics. The lists of the miasmatic connections of the bowel nosodes have been expanded to include the tubercular and cancer miasms. Minor additions to the materia medica of the individual nosodes have been made, and slight changes and additions to the amended associated remedy lists will be found. New cases have been added to some of the previous chapters to illustrate further the usefulness of these unique remedies.

The major change, however, is the creation of an individual chapter for Bacillus No. 10 and hence its removal from the final chapter containing the smaller, in the sense of less frequently indicated, nosodes. This change has been made in the light of the increasing clinical evidence as to the usefulness of this nosode in a number of areas.

Thanks go once more to those professional colleagues who have shared their clinical experiences of using the nosodes and thus helped to broaden further the knowledge of this group of valuable remedies.

PREFACE TO THE THIRD EDITION

An appreciation of the full relationship between the bowel flora and the immune function of the body is necessary for a full understanding of the bowel nosodes. Although there have been sections on this subject in various chapters of the previous editions, in this latest version the opportunity has been taken of pulling these sections together and expanding them to form a new chapter in which the whole subject is discussed more fully.

The whole text has also been revised with additions where appropriate and two further cases have been included. It is hoped that these changes will further enhance the book and that it will continue to be of interest and use to the homeopathic community.

John Saxton
June 1st 2020

ABOUT THE AUTHOR

John Saxton qualified from the Royal Veterinary College in 1964, obtaining his Veterinary Membership of the Faculty of Homeopathy in 1988, and his Veterinary Fellowship in 1996. After nearly forty years in general practice he now runs a veterinary homeopathic referral practice as well as writing, teaching and examining in homeopathy. He lectures nationally and internationally to doctors, veterinary surgeons and nurses, both independently and as part of the Homeopathic Professionals Teaching Group. He is an examiner for the Faculty of Homeopathy and a recognised teacher and examiner for the International Association for Veterinary Homeopathy. He is the author of *Miasms as Practical Tools* and co-author of *Textbook of Veterinary Homeopathy*.

ACKNOWLEDGEMENTS

This book has benefited from the advice of many people. In particular I am grateful to Dr Raymond Sevar and Francis Treuherz who have read the manuscript, made many useful suggestions, and kindly allowed me access to some of their copyright material. I was also extremely fortunate that Geoffrey Brown passed on to me his copies of many of the major articles on the bowel nosodes which contain, where appropriate, hand written notes from his conversations with Dr John Paterson. Geoffrey Brown of Bradford, a Tax Consultant was a personal friend of Drs John and Elizabeth Paterson, to whom he was introduced through his father's interest in homeopathy, and who allowed the Paterson's to use part of their house as consulting rooms twice a week. During the fifties and sixties, Geoffrey was a frequent visitor to the Faculty in London. Thanks are also due to Dr Peter Fisher, who was editor of the journal *Homeopathy* (formally the *British Homeopathic Journal*) until he was tragically killed in a road accident in 2018, for his kind permission to reproduce passages from that publication. In addition, my colleagues when I was in general practice deserve my thanks, not only for their general support and friendship, but also for their input into some of the cases presented. I am indebted to those of my relatives and friends who have allowed me to use their case in this book. As always, I am immensely grateful to my wife, Pat, firstly for her forbearance when I announced that I was planning to write another book, and also for her subsequent tolerance, active encouragement and advice.

In addition I have been the beneficiary of the efforts and advice of an understanding and supportive publishing team, to whom I extend my warmest thanks.

The publishers would additionally like to acknowledge Ms Deirdre Combrink-Potter, a student of Homeopathy at the Durban University of Technology in South Africa, whose MTech dissertation on the bowel nosodes prompted some useful discussions during the preparation of this 3rd edition.

John Saxton

1

ORIGINS AND DEVELOPMENT

The source

The source materials for the bowel nosodes are certain groups of bacteria that are found as part of the bacterial flora of the human intestine in particular states of ill health, and at specific stages of the disease process. They belong to the group broadly identified as *non-lactose fermenting bacilli* (NLFB), but within that classification individual members were identified specifically by their ability or otherwise to ferment three other sugars, namely glucose, saccharose and dulcitol. Apart from two of the sub-groups that consist of cocci, all are members of the salmonella and enterobacteria species and, except for one, they are all Gram-negative. Modern bacteriology has changed enormously in respect of both techniques and nomenclature since the days of the early work on the bowel nosodes, and they are now classed as being among the genera Klebsiella, Enterobacter, Serratia, Proteus and others (Cummings 1988). The modern nomenclature is given at the end of this chapter.

The use of lactose as the basis for the classification was purely as a result of standard laboratory protocols, but it must be remembered that lactose is the only sugar of animal origin used as a routine in the laboratory, and it is also the only sugar capable of having a major influence on the composition of the bowel flora. In the first half of the twentieth century, work at Yale established a link between lactose and the influence on the bowel flora of *Bacillus acidophilus* (Rettiger & Cheplin 1921). It was demonstrated in the work that lactose was the only sugar capable of altering the bowel flora in this way, hence its usefulness as an investigative medium. This is discussed further in Chapter 2 in connection with diet, but the subsequent development of *B acidophilus* plus other bacteria and some yeasts as probiotics that encourage and support the body's natural healing potential demonstrates the close connection between the bowel flora and disease states generally.

The laboratory technique involved in the production and identification of the relevant NLFBs was in two stages, and followed the standard identification protocol used for the identification of enterobacteria species that had been devised by MacConkey in the early years of the twentieth century. The initial culture of a faecal swab was on MacConkey agar for eighteen hours at 37.5°C. This stage resulted in the separation of the gram negative and gram positive bacteria. The Gram-negative NLFB thus produced were then incubated again for a further eighteen hours. After this stage the resulting individual colonies were added to one percent solutions of the other three sugars involved in the identification process; the subsequent reactions, in respect of acid and gas formation, determining after another eighteen hours the exact classification. The time element is important as eighteen hours was chosen for the incubation period, rather than the more normal seventy-two hours, because it was shown that variations in the bacteria's fermenting power at that stage were of potential pathogenic significance (Paterson 1949).

Although an essentially simple and straightforward technique, it was found to be important that it was followed exactly, otherwise false results would ensue. After the 9th Quinquennial International Homoeopathic Congress held in London in conjunction with the International Homoeopathic League in 1927, at which the work on the bowel nosodes received major publicity, a number of overseas workers became interested, but failed to obtain satisfactory results. Dr John Paterson (see below) came to the conclusion, following correspondence with them, that their failure to follow the technique faithfully was to blame for their lack of success (Paterson 1936a).

The initial work

The initial work that led ultimately to the development of the remedies took place in the purely conventional field. Over the years the names of several workers have been linked to the bowel nosodes, and although much valuable work has been contributed by several people there are two names of major importance, those of Bach and Paterson. Dr Edward Bach (1886–1936) was the prime mover in the early years, and when he left the field in 1930 to begin his work on the Flower Remedies, Dr John Paterson (1890–1954) and his wife Dr Elizabeth Paterson (1907–1963) in Glasgow carried the work forward. Sometimes the names of the bowel nosodes (see below) are seen associated with one or another of these names, and this is a recognition of the initial work on and definition of the appropriate bacterial group from which the nosode is derived.

It was in 1880 that the first non lactose fermenting bacillus, linked to typhoid, had been isolated by bacteriologist Karl Ebert. Other bacilli of varying degrees of pathogenicity followed without creating too much interest in the medical world. Although Koch (1843–1910) and Loeffler (1852–1915) did not publish the *postulaes*, their definitive statement of Germ Theory until 1884 the idea of causative links between bacteria and specific diseases were current before that time and the lack of interest in the early NLFB was mainly because they could not generally be linked with specific pathological processes. It was not until about 1912, when Dr Bach became interested, that any serious investigation of them took place. At the time Dr Bach was working in the bacteriology department of University College Hospital London, and as a result of his work he came to realise that a number of these non-lactose fermenting, gram negative bacteria, which appeared to be essentially non-pathogenic, had in fact a close connection with chronic disease generally.

The thrust of the conventional work was concerned with the use of autogenous vaccines, based on faecal swabs, in the treatment of chronic disease states. The general principle of vaccination for prophylaxis was, of course, firmly established by this time. Vaccination as a means of treatment was less recognised. In the conventional work, treatment was by way of the injection of vaccines prepared from killed cultures of the bacteria isolated in individual cases. The clinical results were encouraging, but within the thinking of the time, based as it was on germ theory, they were interpreted as indicating that the organisms isolated were implicated in the cause of the presenting disease. The dramatist George Bernard Shaw was a close friend of Dr Almroth Wright, who worked in the immunology department of St Mary's Hospital, London. His portrayal of the conventional medical attitudes of the time, and the public's reaction to them, in Act 1 of his play *The Doctor's Dilemma*, written in 1906, is an interesting reflection of the prevailing social thought patterns of the times.

In 1919, following a severe illness two years previously (at one stage he was given only three months to live), Dr Bach moved from University College Hospital to the Royal London Homoeopathic Hospital (now known as the Royal London Hospital for Integrated Medicine), primarily as a bacteriologist. From his own experience he had become convinced of the importance of the mind in the processes of disease and cure and his full exposure to the philosophy and methodology of homeopathy, which he found to be very much in tune with his own developing concepts of disease. Even as a medical student, and increasingly through his time as an orthodox doctor, he had felt that the key to cure lay in treating the whole patient, particularly regarding their mental aspects, and not just the particular symptoms and organs (Weeks circa 1940). He read the *Organon* with enthusiasm and considered it the work of a genius (Bach 1920).

In 1920 Dr Bach presented a paper entitled *The Relation of Vaccine Therapy to Homoeopathy* to the British Homoeopathic Society, subsequently published in the *British Homeopathic Journal*. In it, though coming from an allopathic background, he states his admiration for Hahnemann's work and for the science of homeopathy in general. His view was that vaccine therapy, as opposed to prophylaxis, was a 'modern branch of medical science extraordinarily closely related to your own methods [homeopathy], and, on account of the good results obtained, may be worthy of consideration as a modern confirmation of the truths of homeopathy'. He stressed the fact that the vaccines used for treatment contained a minimal dose of the bacteria, equivalent to the dilution found round a seven or eight × potency. This was compared with the concentration of bacteria found in prophylactic vaccines, that being up to a thousand times greater. He had also begun to use the vaccines orally in potentised form and found the results to be as good as when they were given in material dose by injection.

In the early days the emphasis of the ideas concerning the NLFB and the autogenous vaccination technique was based round the concept of 'intestinal toxaemia'. In 1925 Drs Bach and Wheeler published *Chronic Disease: a Working Hypothesis* in which they expanded on this. In essence, chronic disease was held to be caused by the absorption of toxins from the bowels, to a greater or lesser degree depending on the permeability of the individual intestinal mucosa. Modern thought is in terms of alimentary immunity rather than simple permeability. The toxins were thought to be produced by the NLFB with the presence of these latter being due primarily to dietary factors. Hence great store was laid on dietary changes for the patient, especially concerning an increase in the proportion of raw food in the diet. As a result of conventional experience, the vaccination regime that was employed followed the homeopathic usage, with the dose not being repeated automatically at a set interval, but rather according to the clinical condition of the patient (Bach 1928). Nevertheless, the overall view expressed in the book was still governed by the 'cause and effect' thinking of the orthodox approach.

In 1924 an observation was reported by Dr Wheeler that is of such crucial importance to the understanding of the bowel nosodes that it and some subsequent reports warrant quoting verbatim.

In his paper *A New Nosode* he states:

> For days together Dr Bach made faecal examinations and discovered a most interesting phenomenon. When a chronic case gives a positive faecal result it is quite common for the colonies of the presumed offender to number only 2 to 5 percent or even less of the faecal flora. Treat most cases successfully, either with a vaccine, a potentised nosode or the indicated remedy (and in all our cases whenever we

were reasonably sure of it we preferred the indicated remedy) and at once the percentage goes up till the organism may be obtained in all but pure culture. This *only* happens if the case improves and *always* happens if the case improves, whatever the curative remedy. . . .

The use of the phrase 'presumed offender' in the above is interesting and gives an indication of the conventional thought pattern that was still influencing the work.

Dr Wheeler then goes on to emphasis the positive nature of this reaction, and the large numbers of NLFB that accompany it, in contrast to the negative stage of the disease in which only small numbers of NLFB, or none at all, are found. Later in the article he states further that as the case progresses towards cure, the colonies, at first so strikingly increased, gradually lessen, and when they disappear the cure is complete.'

It is in this same article that Wheeler reports Dr Bach's belief that intestinal toxaemia is synonymous with psora, the most basic of the miasms as described by Hahnemann, with which opinion he agreed. He cites in support the 'profound abdominal symptoms' that are to be found in all the major antipsoric remedies. In 1928 Dr Bach presented his paper *The Rediscovery of Psora* (published 1929) to the British Homoeopathic Society in which he reiterates this view, but in which he states much more. Building on Dr Wheeler's comments in 1924 he expands on the positive and negative stages of chronic disease. It had been found by continuous culture of faecal samples from patients that the NLFB:

> . . . are not persistently and constantly present, but that there are negative phases when they are entirely absent, and positive ones when they are present in varying proportions. Moreover, the total numbers during the positive phases vary from day to day. If we start plating [culturing] during a negative phase, after a time they begin to appear in the specimens, at first in small numbers, then steadily rising each day until the maximum is reached when the percentage again falls until they disappear.

Although it was found that there could be considerable variation in the length of the two phases in individual cases, it had become clear that:

> . . . the health of the individual, whether in disease or in an apparently normal condition, varies directly with these phases. Most commonly in cases of chronic disease the symptoms are worse towards the end of the negative period. . . .

Confirmation of these results was coming from similar work by Drs William Boyd and John Paterson in Glasgow, who were further exploring the same issues, and five weeks after the above paper was presented Dr Paterson presented his *Psora in Children and the Use of the Bach Nosodes* to the Society (published 1929).

It is interesting to note from Dr Bach's paper that the value of the homeopathic method of only giving doses (in their case of vaccine) when 'clinically indicated' rather than 'at regular intervals' had been appreciated independently during his time at University College Hospital. Initially this had been noted in cases of acute febrile disease, particularly pneumonia, but later in chronic disease also. As a rule of thumb, doses of vaccine in chronic disease were never repeated in less than three weeks as it had been found that on occasion it required this length of time for an improvement to begin. It was facts such as this that, on subsequently reading the *Organon*, led him to state:

> On reading Hahnemann's *Organon* for the first time one instantly recognises the fact that the work of the modern immunity school was merely the rediscovery, by a different method, of facts that had been realised by him a century before. . . .

The dosage observations noted above would indicate the possibility of some active reaction on the part of the patient being involved in the response to treatment. In addition, by this time Dr Bach was moving from the original orthodox view of the NLFBs. In 1925 he had written 'Results (from his injectable vaccines) are so striking that it is very difficult to resist the conviction that the organisms are related to the disease as cause and effect' (Land 2008). He had then moved from that view within the causative format to a position where he was wondering:

> . . . whether these organisms are the cause, the result or an attempted cure of disease.

Another indication of Bach's line of thinking is contained in his comment that 'I wish it were possible that we could present to you seven herbs instead of seven groups of bacteria because there always seems to be some reticence in the minds of many to use anything associated with disease in the treatment of pathological conditions' (Bach 1928). At that time only seven of the final thirteen groups of bacteria in use today had been identified, and at one stage Dr Bach considered that seven was the total number, equating them with the seven basic personality types that he had identified. Even when he had developed his full range of thirty-eight Flower Remedies he still classified them into the seven groups representing what he saw as the basic overriding emotional states of man, namely fear, uncertainty, disinterest, loneliness, over sensitivity, despondency and over concern for others. Although at the time he wrote his comment he was undoubtedly reflecting the debate that was current among those working in the field as to the pathogenicity or otherwise of the bacteria involved, it is likely that he felt the dilemma more keenly than most as it was only some two years later that he quit both his practice and research activities and commenced his search for his Flower Remedies.

Further development

It was at this point that the emphasis of the work shifted to Glasgow, although, as has been indicated above, a team there was already involved in the field. At the Scottish Homoeopathic Hospital for Children, later to become the Glasgow Homoeopathic Hospital, Dr Thomas Dishington, as clinical head, conceived the idea of using the nosodes of Dr Bach in potentised form, and it was from this that Dr John Paterson began his major involvement in the early months of 1927. With this move to Glasgow the further development of the work was fixed firmly within the homeopathic ethos, in contrast to the work of Edward Bach, who came from a non homeopathic background. Dr John Paterson was also a bacteriologist and although both he and his wife were meticulous researchers, they were primarily practicing physicians and hence their work was always directed by extensive clinical observations on a broad front. In 1928 Dr John Paterson had presented his paper on psora in children, much of which consisted of case reports. However, in the first part he explores the limitations of classical germ theory and the role of host susceptibility in disease, as well as suggesting links between the bowel nosodes and Hahnemann's three basic miasms of psora, sycosis and syphilis. In the paper, *Psora in children and the use of the Bach nosodes,* he is concerned primarily, as its title suggests, with the treatment of psoric manifestations using Dr Bach's nosodes, appreciating the position of the miasm as the 'soil' into which disease implants. He also interprets Dr Bach's work as indicating the association of particular pathological changes with the presence of certain specific bacteria. However, it is clear that he also had an understanding of the role of all the three basic miasms in chronic disease and considered it likely that there were further groups of NLFB connected to the other miasms.

Dr Paterson, of course, viewed chronic disease from the point of view of a homeopath, outlining that view in his introductory address to students at the Royal London Homoeopathic Hospital. He described chronic disease as being deep seated within the body, capable of producing a wide range of symptoms and potentially involving more than one system (Paterson 1933a). In his address to the Scottish branch of the Faculty of Homoeopathy in 1953 he reiterates the sense in which Hahnemann uses the term 'chronic' as denoting the depth of action of disease rather than the length of time it had been present. In many cases time is inevitably a factor but not the essence of the condition.

Meanwhile, other workers had identified and described other groups of NLFB. Dr Wheeler in his paper of 1924 outlined the clinical aspects of another group linked to Dr Bach's work but without the close connection to the psoric miasm, while in 1929 Dr Dishington had published a paper on the pathogenesis of dysentery and identified NLFBs associated with the condition. In this he states that 'Disease is not an entity to be expelled from the body, but a dynamic error in the life forces, an unbalance in the vital functions that can be corrected only by the recuperative power within the living cells themselves' and also that 'the bacteria cannot be looked upon as the sole causation of the disease, but are present because of the dynamic error within the life of the patient'.

The miasmatic connection of the bowel nosodes was further emphasised in a paper by John Paterson dealing with the development of another group of bacteria with a definite relationship to sycosis (Paterson 1933b). In this paper he questions the interpretation of Dr Tyler in her *Hahnemann's Conception of Chronic Disease, as Caused by Parasitic Micro-organisms* (1933) as leaning too much towards the germ theory approach of the orthodox school, and contrasts this with what he saw as Hahnemann's view of miasms as a more functional balance involving micro-organisms as part of the dynamic picture but without the causal link. He also answers Dr Bach's query as to the role of the NLFB in disease by stating that:

> The non-lactose organisms found in the bowel are the result of a vital reaction on the part of the body tissues.

In this statement the term 'vital' is being used in the Hahnemannian sense of a living reaction within the context of a healing process.

In 1936 Paterson presented his paper *The Potentised Drug and its Action on the Bowel Flora*, in which he amplified his thoughts, stating that 'The appearance of non-lactose fermenting organisms I regard as evidence of the action of the action of the defensive body mechanism'. This paper was based on his observations over some eight years and contains several points of major interest. The first of these concerned the early stages of his work, when, after a few months he visited the workers in London and compared the results of his cultures with those being obtained by the southern team. To his consternation it transpired that there were significant differences between the two. The Glasgow findings were producing a greater number of positive results for NLFB than were apparent in London. After checking the standardisation of the culture technique and other factors, there appeared to be only one possible explanation for this, which lay in the different nature of the patients presenting at the two centres. In London the bulk of patients from whom faecal swabs were taken had, prior to their involvement, been treated by their orthodox allopathic doctors. In contrast, those at Glasgow were almost entirely drawn from a group who had been under the care of homeopathic doctors. Hence these patients had received homeopathic remedies as their main form of treatment. This fact immediately raised the question as to whether homeopathic remedies were capable of changing the bowel flora, and after his years of experience John Paterson's conclusion was that they did. In his paper *The Role of the Bowel Flora in Chronic Disease* (1949) he presented what he described as 'twenty years observations as physician and bacteriologist' and offered an explanation as to the possible mode of action of the observed bowel changes (see below).

Other points worthy of attention are the observation that there is always a 'latent period' following the administration of a remedy before any NLFBs are found in the stool. This is generally between ten and fourteen days, an interval familiar to medicine in other clinical reactions such as vaccination. Occasionally it is of much shorter duration, around three days, but that is uncommon. When that does occur it is seen either in children where any potency may have been employed, or in adults where high potencies had been used. Dr Paterson considered that the shorter the latent period following the administration of a remedy, the nearer to the apparent worsening of a therapeutic aggravation the patient had been pushed. He considered the ideal response to be one that occurred after ten days, producing not too great a percentage of NLFB, and passing off in a reasonable period of time. What was considered reasonable varied with the level of disease present. It is interesting to note that modern clinical experience is that improvement in the condition of the patient is frequently seen before any changes in the bowel flora would be expected, sometimes within twenty four hours. (See Chapter 4 for discussion of potency considerations with the bowel nosodes.)

Experience also revealed high variability in both the percentage and duration of the NLFBs in the individual stools. The percentage in different cases was found to range from one to one hundred, and similarly the period of its presence could be from a few days to a few months.

1949 saw the publication of two more papers by John Paterson. In the first, *The Role of the Bowel Flora in Chronic Disease* he cites five hundred cases where a polyvalent vaccine of all types of NLFB was administered by injection, resulting in 95% showing a definite beneficial effect with 80% being good to excellent. He also offers a possible explanation of the mechanism of the bowel nosode reaction. His hypothesis was based on the idea that bacteria will mutate in order to survive in the environment in which they find themselves: he considered that the administration of a remedy to a patient would set in motion various chemical changes in the cells, and these would have an impact on the enzymes of the bowel mucosa, which would in turn affect the environment in which the bowel bacteria were living. These would then adapt in order to survive. Continuing improvement in the patient's health would be mirrored by further metabolic changes, inducing at the end of the chain other changes in the bowel flora.

The second paper from 1949, *The Bowel Nosodes*, was presented at the International Homoeopathic League Council in Lyon in August, subsequently being published as a pamphlet which is still available. It is very much a clinical guide to eight of the bowel nosodes, encompassing materia medica and instructions on the use of the agents in the disease situation. It does however also contain a brief review of the conclusions drawn from the work to date, with the emphasis on two points. Firstly that the NLFB in a case, although possibly veering towards the pathogenic, are not in any way the cause of the disease. Dr Paterson himself preferred in fact to use the term 'pathogenic' as implying being linked to disease rather than the more accepted usage of causing disease. The second point was that the appearance of the bacteria occurs following the administration of a correctly selected homeopathic remedy and a resultant improvement in the patients wellbeing. He was thus able to state that:

(a) The specific organism is related to the disease.
(b) The specific organism is related to the homeopathic remedy.
(c) The homeopathic remedy is related to the disease.

This may be represented by an equilateral triangle:

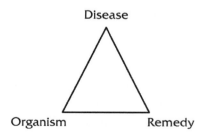

This paper marked the end of the period of extensive research work on the bowel nosodes. A major factor in this decline was the advent of the chemically-based therapeutic era with the consequent major and widespread disturbances in the bowel flora that ensued. As might be expected, anti-biotics had a profound effect, but other agents such as steroids also played their part. In 1949 Paterson published the results of work into a variation of the basic Bach nosode linked to the remedy Lycopodium and in 1954 Dr Kennedy reported on the results of a series of three hundred and twenty three cases involving various conditions and medications over a three year period where faecal swabs were used as part of the investigative method. These were split into both control and treatment groups (termed 'provers' in the article) and provided further insights into the percentages of NLFB that might be expected in practice. Although there were variations between the nosode groups, it was demonstrated overall that the drug administration had a definite effect in changing the makeup of the bowel flora. Apart from those the other major contribution was from Dr Elizabeth Paterson who published *A Survey of the Nosodes* (1960) that provided a valuable review of three hundred and thirty consecutive and unselected cases involving the clinical application of the bowel nosodes.

The eleven bowel nosodes that were finally described are Morgan Pure, Morgan Gaertner, Dysentery Co, Proteus, Sycotic Co, Gaertner Bach, Bacillus No 7, Bacillus No 10, Mutabile, Faecalis and Coccal Co. The remedy Morgan Bach is often used in practice and is a combination of Morgan Pure and Morgan Gaertner (see Chapter 5 for details). The designation 'Co' in this context stands for compound, implying the presence of several bacterial strains in the source material of each remedy. Each of the bowel nosodes is based on polyvalent cultures from multiple patients exhibiting the same range of symptoms. A combination of all the nosodes except Sycotic Co has also been used under the name of, initially, 'P.B.V.' but being known latterly as 'PolyBowel (Bach)'.

Various commentaries and critiques of the bowel nosodes have appeared over the years (Gordon Ross 1973; Cummings 1988; Neustaedter 1988; Laing 1995). Neustaedter in his *Critique of the Bowel Nosodes* raised several major objections to the whole concept, and it is pertinent to address his concerns. He based his criticism in large part on the fact that no provings in the full Hahnemannian tradition have been carried out on any of the bowel nosodes. This criticism was raised in the very early days of the bowel nosodes and had been addressed by Dr Paterson. In 1929 he pointed out that the traditional homeopathic method of building up a drug picture employed not only provings on healthy subjects, but also made use of material based on clinical observations in cases of disease. In 1936 he stated that drug pictures for the nosodes could by built by accurate observation of clinical symptoms and verified by comparison with the known drug pictures of the remedies that had been shown to be associated with the various nosodes. (See Chapter 2 for a full discussion of the associated remedies.) Neustaedter however concludes from the lack of traditional provings that 'most of the research on bowel nosodes is based on theory'. Whilst it is true that no formal provings have been carried out, to the author this argument appears disingenuous. Neustaedter himself acknowledges that 'It is not terribly unusual in homeopathy to use drugs that have no provings' and cites Symphytum, Kali Sulphuricum and 'several other nosodes' as examples, saying 'We have these precedents for prescribing on the basis of anecdotal clinical data exclusively, but the presence of provings is always reassuring and welcome.' Whilst no one would question the usefulness of traditional provings, doubt has been cast of the reliability of many of them, and attention has been drawn to their tendency to over-estimate the number of meaningful symptoms produced (Dantas 2007). In both the *Organon* (Paragraph 136) and the preface to *Materia Medica Pura* (1830) Hahnemann recognises the value of symptoms obtained from clinical experience. Prior to that, in his *Essay on a New Principle for Ascertaining the Curative Power of Drugs* (1796) he rates 'observations of its (the medicine's) action in this or that simple or complex disease' on a par with 'the pure action of each (medicine) by itself on the human body'. Bearing in mind that Hahnemann was unlikely to have envisaged the development and usage of bacteriology in modern medicine at this time, his statement represents, to the author, a clear endorsement of the value of clinical observation and investigation alongside formal provings. Hence it is a long way from provings being 'reassuring and welcome' to the stance that nothing should be prescribed without their backup, which is what Neustaedter appears to be implying should be the case for assessing the bowel nosodes, and apparently for them alone. He also states 'The only way besides provings to establish indications for any medicine is to formulate a theory and attempt to verify it through experimentation', but the fact of the variable presence of NLFB in the bowels during illness has never been questioned and the theories that emerged to explain that have, over a number of decades, been developed into a practical and useful clinical method. Nor is it the case today that there is a dearth of clinical material to support the materia medica of the nosodes. The drug pictures of the bowel nosodes are already significant and are constantly growing. Whilst accepting the possibility that Paterson's explanation of NLFB stimulation during healing is correct, he states 'to base a prescription on such convoluted theoretical assumptions is certainly not consistent with Hahnemannian principles', but Hahnemann's basic principle of observation and experiment has been followed faithfully throughout the work.

Neustaedter's remarks about John Paterson's caution with regard to his instructions for use fail to take account of the fact that they were written during the development of the remedies and make no allowance for the clinical experience that has been acquired since then. Similarly the point about Dr Bach's 'metaphysical penchant for numerology in medicine' appears irrelevant. Whatever the reason, Bach's opinion that there were only seven bowel nosodes was clearly incorrect and that view had no influence on the situation there is today as he left the work before the major clinical development of the concept.

A more serious point is the one he shares with Cummings (1988) regarding the uncertainties of the bacteriology associated with the bowel nosodes. Bacteriological techniques have certainly advanced since the early part of the twentieth century and those employed in the original work would not be considered adequate today. Not only that, but the terminology and classification have also changed in line with new knowledge. This undoubtedly gives potential problems for the compilers of pharmacopoeia and the manufacturing pharmacies with regard to quality control, especially in relation to some of the clinical entities (see below). Currently bowel nosodes do not feature in the pharmacopoeias that form the basis of the standards for remedy production. However, it has been possible to make some comparisons and express the composition of most of the nosodes in modern terms (Alexander 1988). That classification, as listed below, was used as the basis of identification during investigation of the similarities or otherwise between the original findings in humans and the situation that exists in certain animal species (Saxton 1994). The confluence between the results, although far from absolute proof of the correctness of the modern equivalence, may possibly be interpreted as indicating a degree of accuracy. (See Chapter 2 for discussion of this work.)

It cannot be denied that this area represents a definite gap in the overall bowel nosode picture that is particularly galling from the perspective of pure bacteriology. More work certainly needs to be done on this aspect. The currently available remedies are based on historical sources, and Paterson's originals are still in use. Any recreation of them from modern sources would be virtually impossible as a result of both the prevalence of antibiotics in the human alimentary system and the generally suppressive emphasis of current treatment methods. Even if such a recreation was possible, it would have to take account of the reclassification issue, and also address the possibility of mutation (Kayne L 2006). However, it must be remembered that the bowel nosodes as clinical entities have a well proven and established clinical record on which prescription may be made with confidence. It must also be stressed that the supply of the bowel nosodes is in no way threatened and supplies of basic potencies are more than adequate.

The relationship to modern bacteriology

Each of the bowel nosodes represents a group of bacteria, hence the references to 'polyvalent vaccines' that are found in the original papers. At the present time, unfortunately, it has not been possible to identify the modern equivalents of some of the clinical entities, notably Gaertner Bach and Bacillus No 10, and equally the position regarding Coccal Co is not completely clear.

Morgan Pure

Morganella morganii, Proteus mirabilis, Aeromonas salmonicida, Salmonella subgenus IV, Edwardsiella tarda, Escherichia blattae, Hafnia alvei.

Morgan Gaertner

Salmonella paratyphi A, S. subgenus 2&3, Salmonella cholersuis.

Proteus

Edwardsiella hoshinae, Edwardsiella tarda biogroup 1, Obesumbacterium proteus biogroup 2, Proteus myxofaciens, Proteus penneri, Proteus vulgaris biogroup 2.

Dysentery Co

Shigella dysenteriae, Shigella flexneri, Shigella boydii, Salmonella gallinarum, Salmonella typhisus.

Sycotic Co

Streptococcus faecalis, Acinetobacter calcoaeticus lwoffii.

Bacillus No 7

Citrobacter koseri, Enterobacter cloacae.

Mutabile

Morganella morganii, Salmonella subgenus 3.

Faecalis

Alcaligenes faecalis.

Coccal Co

A number of gram-positive bowel cocci.

2

THE PRACTICAL IMPLICATIONS

The associated remedies

Various relationships between homeopathic remedies are well recognised and used in clinical practice. One such relationship is the idea of 'acute' and 'chronic' remedies, for example that 'Silica is the chronic of Pulsatilla' or 'Bryonia is the acute of Natrum Muriaticum'; meaning that where the one is used successfully to treat disease at one level, the related remedy will be generally be useful to treat disease at the other level in the same patient (by implication, Pulsatilla is also the acute of Silica and Natrum Muriaticum is the chronic of Bryonia). Other relationships involve remedies that either 'follow well', 'complement' or 'antidote' each other and those that are inimical (incompatible). Desirable and effective prescribing sequences such as Calcarea Carbonica followed by Lycopodium followed by Sulphur or Sulphur moving to Sarsaparilla and then on to Sepia have been identified also (Blasig and Vint 2001).

In the author's opinion, the connection between the bowel nosodes and other remedies is of an entirely different nature to any of the above. In all those relationships outlined above, the effect is essentially one of a remedy either interfering with or building on the action of another; the actions are separate and sequential. The positive inter-action between a bowel nosode and a remedy is of a more synergistic nature and is often contemporaneous. Hence the term 'associated remedies' is preferable in their context (see Chapter 4 for the clinical applications of the bowel nosodes). The term 'related' is still widely used; on occasion 'indicated' will be seen, and all are referring to the same thing, but the two latter terms do not accurately reflect the unique position of the bowel nosodes.

As has been shown in Chapter 1, it was found that the application of a correct treatment to a patient resulted in an improvement in the wellbeing of that patient, accompanied by the appearance in the stool of significant numbers of NLFB. In the initial stages of the work, as mentioned, treatments were by injection of vaccines produced from the individual stools of patients. The use of potentised vaccines was added later but whilst the focus of the development remained in London there were different types of treatment being administered to patients. With the move to Glasgow, however, the treatments became entirely homeopathic, with the remedies being selected in line with the classical tradition of homeopathy.

It became clear that not only were well selected remedies producing improvement in the patients linked to the appearance of NLFB in the stools, but that different remedies caused different groups of the bacteria to be found in the stool. It was also observed that, across the range of patients, if the same remedy was indicated and proved successful, then consistently the same NLFB would become present in the stool. It is interesting to note how aware John Paterson was of the risk of personal bias coming into the interpretation of his results, since he was both physician and bacteriologist for many of the cases in the hospital. He accordingly utilised the findings obtained from faecal samples that were submitted by homeopathic colleagues and found that he was able to work out from the results of a sample what remedy had been given previously. Alternatively, knowing what remedy had been given to a patient, he was able to predict accurately the type of NLFB that would subsequently be found in the stool (Paterson 1936).

John Paterson had defined the relationship between the disease, the organism and the remedy in his paper to the International Homeopathic League in 1949 (see Chapter 1). Because of the homeopathic method of remedy selection, this could also be expressed as:

Symptom Picture

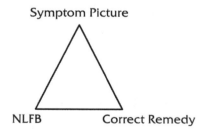

NLFB   Correct Remedy

It will be appreciated that because, in the clinical situation, the correct remedy is connected to the symptom picture, and also that successful treatment establishes a link between that remedy and the particular NLFB, there is consequently a relationship between the symptom picture and the appearing bacteria.

The first definite pattern of a relationship between a remedy and a group of NLFB was that between Natrum Muriaticum and B. Proteus. The next stage in his thinking was hence couched in relation to these two. *The*

Potentised Drug and its Action on the Bowel Flora (1936) he discussed how several cases presenting with little clinical data had revealed B. Proteus in their pre-treatment faecal samples. This caused him to pose the question: 'If Nat Mur causes B. Proteus to appear in the stool, may not this remedy be efficacious in the patient yielding B. Proteus in high percentage?'

This hypothesis was tested with appropriate clinical cases, not only involving Natrum Muriaticum and B. Proteus but also with other cases yielding other groups of NLFB. Following the successful verification of this idea, the triangle above was able to be adapted to:

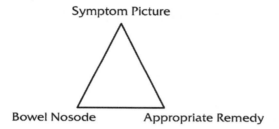

It is the interrelationship represented by this triangle that forms the basis for the concept of the associated remedies. Based on clinical observations, lists of remedies were drawn up detailing their connection to the various individual bowel nosodes. These lists are given below and represent the clinical experience of the major original workers in the field.

It will be noted that in the lists the remedies are designated in the same way as is standard in all repertories, namely bold type, italics or plain type. This indicates the closeness of the link that has been established, with the remedies in bold type being those that would regularly stimulate the production of appropriate NLFB in significant numbers. Such a bold type remedy is referred to as a 'leading remedy' of that group. However, it must be remembered that with all the listed remedies a definite link has been established, and it is a mistake to concentrate exclusively on the bold type entries. It will also be seen that some remedies are represented in more than one group, but as far as the highest designation of bold type is concerned, the remedy will only ever appear in one group at that level. The presence of a leading remedy of one group at a lower grading in the associated list of another nosode indicates a degree of overlap in the symptom picture of the remedy in relation to the respective nosodes. As far as the italic and plain type entries are concerned, in clinical terms this means that using the nosode associated with the remedy concerned will result in definite benefit to some part of the symptom picture but the whole clinical picture may not be covered.

The traditionally associated remedy lists (Paterson 1949)

Morgan Pure

Alumina, Baryta Carb, Calc Carb, Calc Sulph, Carbo Veg, Carbo Sulph, Digitalis Purp, Ferrum Carb, *Graphites*, Kali Carb, Mag Carb, *Medorrhinum*, Natrum Carb, Petroleum, *Psorinum*, Sepia Off, **Sulphur**, Tuberculinum Bov.

Morgan Gaertner

Chelidonium Maj, Chenopodium Ant, Helleborus Niger, Hepar Sulph, *Lachesis Muta*, **Lycopodium Clav**, Merc Sulph, Sanguinaria Can, Taraxacum Off.

Proteus

Acid Mur, Ammonium Mur, Aurum Mur, Apis Mel, Baryta Mur, Borax, Calc Mur, Conium Mac, Cuprum Met, Ferrum Mur, Ignatia Amara, Kali Mur, Mag Mur, **Natrum Mur**, Secale Corn.

Mutabile

Ferrum Phos, Kali Phos, Kali Sulph, **Pulsatilla Nig**.

Gaertner Bach

Calc Fluor, Calc Hypophos, Calc Phos, Calc Sil, Kali Phos, **Merc Viv**, Natrum Phos, Natrum Silicofluor, **Phosphorus**, Phytolacca Dec, Pulsatilla Nig, **Silicea**, Syphilinum, Zinc Phos.

Dysentery Co

Anacardium Or, Argent Nit, **Arsenicum Alb**, Cadmium Met, Kalmia Lat, Veratrum Alb, Veratrum Vir.

Bacillus No. 7

Arsenicum Iod, *Bromium*, Calc Iod, Ferrum Iod, **Iodum**, Kali Bich, Kali Brom, **Kali Carb**, Kali Nit, Merc Iod, Natrum Iod.

Faecalis

Sepia Off.

Sycotic Co

Acid Nit, Antimonium Tart, Bacillinum, Calcium Metal*, Ferrum Met, Natrum Sulph, Rhus Tox, *Thuja Occ*.

*It is unclear what is meant by this entry in Paterson's list but it is included for completeness.

Bacillus No 10
Calc Fluor.

Coccal Co
Tuberculinum Bov.

No or unidentified growth
Merc Sol, Tuberculinum Bov.

It must be remembered that the lists are not necessarily closed and that the above are only an expression of the accepted clinical knowledge in relation to the bowel nosodes up to the end of the period in which the major work was carried out. Many new remedies have entered the materia medica since the 1940s and clinical experience has resulted in further expansion of the lists. As mentioned in Chapter 1, many modern drugs can have profound effects on the bowel flora, and also on the whole healing dynamic. Such treatments leading to the suppression of disease are much more common today than previously (Saxton 2006). Whilst this does not in any way render the bowel nosodes invalid for the treatment of disease, it does mean that often the traditional 'before and after' technique for taking faecal swabs as a research tool is no longer possible. The most likely source of any future additions to the lists will be clinical experience. Handwritten notes by Geoffrey Brown on his copy of the Lyon 1949 paper indicate that Bacillinum should be added to the unidentified list. John Paterson also included it in his list for Coccal Co in 1948, while presenting to the British Homeopathic Congress in Glasgow. In that same paper John Paterson also lists Merc Sol. as being indicated when no NLFB growth is found, and rates it as a major remedy in that context. Dr Kennedy states the same in his 1954 paper. Dr Gordon Ross (1973) quotes Elizabeth Paterson's experience that the four most indicated remedies in the Morgan Pure group are, in order, Sulphur, Pulsatilla, Graphites and Sepia, but adds that in his experience Sepia is the second most commonly prescribed remedy. In line with that, from clinical experience the author considers that Sepia should be listed in italics in that group. The remedy 'SSC', consisting of Sulphur, Silica and Carbo Vegetabilis together appears to act as one compound in the same way that many remedies of plant origin are in fact technically mixtures of several other remedies – such as Lycopodium with its major constituents of Alumina and Silica (Saxton and Gregory 2005). It was at one time in regularly human use for septic conditions, and is still used in the veterinary world, specifically for mastitis. It was included for a while in the associated list for Morgan Pure by Dr Elizabeth Paterson, but has subsequently been dropped from the commonly quoted lists although it is still included in some (Julian 1995). Gunpowder is another remedy mentioned by John Paterson as being possibly associated with the Morgan group that has never appeared in that list. He also expressed the probability that Lycopodium represented part of the Dysentery Co. remedy picture (1949), and stated that Nat Sulph. and Thuja had a close connection to Bacillus No. 10 (1936). It is unfortunately unclear from the literature which form of Merc Iod. is associated with Bacillus No 7, or whether it applies to both.

The appendix contains expanded lists of the associated remedies that are the result of clinical thought and experience since the time the original work was done. The lists included at the start of the chapters on the individual bowel nosodes represent only the accepted and established remedies derived from the original work.

Chemical and other connections of the associated lists

Looking at the lists above, it will be seen that there are various chemical patterns in them, and that both anions and cations may be involved. Both carbon and the carbonates and sulphur and its salts feature largely in the Morgan Pure group, and also to a lesser extent in Morgan Gaertner. John Paterson was of the view that both carbon and sulphur had a role in shaping the characteristics of the two groups (1953). Proteus contains many remedies having a major chlorine component. The group includes many of the major remedies for sadness or grief. That theme fits with the essence of chlorine as envisaged by Jan Scholten in his *Homeopathy and the Elements*, whilst other associated remedies reflect the control and lack of control represented in the group. Bacillus No. 7 reflects the influence of potassium and the weakness associated with the Kali remedies. In the case of Kali Carb. it is present in the first degree in the Morgan Pure group due to the presence of the carbonate, but the effect of the potassium is to raise it to a leading remedy of the Bacillus No. 7 group. Physiologically, potassium has its main influence on the soft tissues of the body rather than the fluids, in contrast to sodium, which is its physiological opposite. However, such is the nature of the halogens that bromine, and especially iodine, exert an effect on the Bacillus No.7 group. Bacillus No 10 has a connection with the other homeopathically relevant halogen, namely fluorine.

Although there is no obvious chemical link in the case of Dysentery Co., a functional link exists via the anxiety that, in some form or other, is present in the picture of many of the remedies. Gaertner Bach has Phosphorus as one of its leading remedies and the phosphates are well represented in the remedy group.

The miasmatic connections

From the early days when Dr Bach first introduced the idea of the connection between intestinal toxaemia and psora, the miasms have been a major part of the bowel nosode story. In his *Hahnemann's Doctrine of Psora and the Homoeopathic Treatment of Skin Disease* (1953), John Paterson stated 'in the treatment of chronic disease which one meets with in practice, it is well nigh impossible to get successful results without a full knowledge of the Hahnemannian doctrine of the miasms, so that one may indeed choose the most similar medicine possible'. The bowel nosodes are both long- and deep-acting remedies and the major indications for their use are found in cases of chronic disease. Their ability to get to the heart of a case is directly linked to the fact that they resonate with the underlying miasmatic pattern of the 'dis-ease'. In Paragraph 204 of the *Organon* Hahnemann emphasised the central role of the miasms in chronic disease. John Paterson (1953) paraphrased the relevant passages of the *Organon* as 'Chronic diseases are caused by dynamic infection with a chronic miasm'. Following Hahnemann's usage, 'infection' was not being applied in this passage in the modern sense of an invasive agent, but rather to indicate a 'disturbance'. Following this line of thought, Paterson agreed with Bach in regard to the connection of Morgan Bach (the original Bach nosode) to the psoric miasm (1929) and also identified a close link between the sycotic miasm and the bowel nosode that he named Sycotic Co. (1933).

These two, however, are not the only miasmatic connections found with the bowel nosodes, and other links are detailed below. The same three-degree grading format as is followed in the repertories is again employed. It will be noted that some of the nosodes appear in more than one of the miasmatic groups, and this reflects the fact that, in common with all other homeopathic remedies, each of the bowel nosodes contains within its make-up elements of all three basic miasms (Saxton 2006). The exact grading given to each nosode reflects the strength of the individual miasmatic influence in that nosode. Thus Morgan Pure is in the third degree in relation to the psoric miasm and also in the second degree for the sycotic miasm: this is mirrored in the associated remedy list by the presence of the major skin remedies such as Sulphur, Graphites, Psorinum and various carbonates providing a psoric connection, while at the same time Medorrhinum and Sepia are represented. Remedies such as Calc Carb. and Baryta

Carb. show clear features of both miasms in their remedy pictures. Likewise the influence of both sycosis and syphilis may be seen within other groupings. Equally, the chemical connections within the groups may indicate some of the miasmatic influences within individual nosodes, such as the psoric weakness of potassium in Bacillus No. 7 and the syphilitic tendency of fluorine in Bacillus No. 10.

The tubercular and cancer miasms have their major representation through the three basic miasms of which they consist but the fixed nature of their miasmatic balance (Saxton 2006) means that they too have their individual connections to the bowel nosodes.

PSORA

Bacillus No. 7; Dysentery Co.; Gaertner Bach; *Morgan Gaertner*; **Morgan Pure**; Mutabile; *Proteus.*

SYCOSIS

Bacillus No. 7; *Bacillus No. 10*; Coccal Co; *Dysentery Co*; *Faecalis*; *Morgan Gaertner*; *Morgan Pure*; *Mutabile*; **Proteus**; **Sycotic Co.**

SYPHILIS

Bacillus No. 7; *Bacillus No. 10*; Dysentery Co.; *Coccal Co.*; **Gaertner Bach**; Proteus.

TUBERCULAR

Bacillus No 7; *Gaertner Bach*; Morgan Pure; Mutabile; *Sycotic Co.*

CANCER

Bacillus No 10; Dysentery Co.; Faecalis; *Gaertner Bach.*

The totality of symptoms

In Paragraph 18 of the *Organon* Hahnemann states 'It is an undeniable truth that nothing can, by any means, be discovered in diseases whereby they could express their need for aid besides the totality of symptoms . . .', and concludes with '. . . the complex of all the symptoms and circumstances perceived in each individual case must be the *only indicator*, the only reference in choosing a remedy'.

Hahnemann wrote both the *Organon* and his other great work, *Chronic Diseases,* before the advent of the range of the modern diagnostic and investigative procedures, but nevertheless his concept encompasses them all. In *Chronic Diseases* he wrote 'To apply successfully the Law of Similars one must find a remedy to cover not only the immediate symptoms of the acute phase [of a chronic condition] but also all the ailments and symptoms inherent in the primitive malady'.

The term 'circumstances' that is used in the first quotation is referenced back by Hahnemann to Paragraph 5 of the *Organon*. In that he lists them, including both lifestyle factors and aspects of the constitutional prescribing with which modern homeopaths are familiar. However, the paragraph ends with 'etc.', and it is not unreasonable to include changes in the disease picture under this cover. Such a change is exactly what the appearance of NLFB represents.

If these two passages are considered together, it will be seen that the bowel nosodes provide a window onto the totality of a case. Chronic disease is a deep and wide- ranging entity, and its symptoms can be equally wide-ranging. Often what is seen on presentation of a case represents, in one sense, only an acute phase of the underlying condition. In many cases, as Hahnemann states in *Chronic Diseases*, successful treatment of that phase does not result in a complete cure (Saxton 2006). It must be remembered that the appearance of NLFB in the stool after the administration of a remedy represents such successful treatment, but without necessarily addressing the complete underlying disturbance. However, the bowel nosode associated with that successful treatment has a connection not only to the remedy given, but also to the other remedies on the appropriate list, which may address in their turn other aspects of the deep problem. That connecting link is manifest in the NLFB produced and hence the bowel nosode, being the remedy based on those bacilli, will address more accurately the true totality of the 'dis-ease' condition than the remedy selected, however accurately, based on only a presenting part of the total picture. It has been said that 'Sadly, the main obstacle to cure remains our inability to get to the core of the case' (Asher 2007), and the use of bowel nosodes offers, in many cases, a possible way round that obstacle.

Are the bowel nosodes truly homeopathic?

This is a question that is still raised by some and has connections to the criticisms of Neustaedter (1988). As discussed in Chapter 1, the essence of this criticism appears to be based around the idea that unless there has been a traditional proving involving healthy human subjects, then a remedy cannot be considered to be indisputably homeopathic. Clinical observation and experience are, if not discounted, then reduced to a supporting role. If this approach is followed too pedantically then many of the newer ways of thinking about remedies, such as those pioneered by the likes of Sherr, Sankaran and Scholten, become invalid. Moreover, as Sherr has demonstrated (2002), there is no intrinsic conflict between these methods and the traditional proving approach, and indeed both can add to a rounded appreciation of a remedy.

In fact, the first ever wonderings about the true nature of the bowel nosodes came from Dr Bach in his address on psora in 1928, and it was in this context that he posed his question regarding 'cause, effect or attempted cure' (see Chapter 1). From the outset he was of the opinion that they were, as he put it 'in accordance with the laws of Hahnemann' and the subsequent clarification of this question by John Paterson confirmed his view. The Drs Paterson were classical in their approach to homeopathy and the sixth edition of the *Organon* was their guide (Brown 1967). In their work it was only the correct remedy that produced both NLFB and an improvement in the patient's condition, the remedy being selected always according to the Law of Similars. In view of the equal relationship that John Paterson demonstrated between the remedy and the nosode, if the one is homeopathic then the other must be also. In his 1949 paper he expresses it as 'The practice of homeopathy is founded on the hypothesis that the true *simillimum* (the homeopathic remedy) is related to the disturbed metabolism (the disease) and now it can be demonstrated that the NLF organism of the bowel is biochemically related to the disease and the homeopathic remedy'. From this he expands the concept of the bowel nosode as a remedy, saying '. . . the nosode, prepared from culture of the organism can be considered to be a complex biochemical substance having the characteristics of the disturbed metabolism, and thus to be similar to the disease and according to the Law of Similars, to have specific therapeutic power to restore balance, a condition of ease – i.e. health'.

Are bowel nosodes true nosodes?

The answer to this question is central to understanding the true nature of the bowel nosodes and their role in treating disease. The term 'nosode' derives from the Greek *nosos* meaning 'disease' and *eides* meaning 'like', and is defined as 'Homeopathic medicine derived from pathological material. May be of human, animal or plant origin, including microorganisms, diseased tissue or the products of disease processes, such as discharges and effusions' (Swayne 2000). 'Pathological' is further defined as 'pertaining to pathology', that is the 'structural and functional changes in tissues and organs of the body which cause or are caused by disease' (Dorland 1974). The confusion arises if a looser definition of a nosode is taken, such as just being a remedy made from 'products of disease' (Vermeulen 2006), and this looser definition is one that is commonly used.

The term 'bowel nosode' was coined at the beginning of the work, and reflected both the then current conventional thought on disease causation and the homeopathic uncertainty as to the true role of the NLFB. Hence it was perhaps inevitable that the terminology being applied to agents such as Diphtherinum, Medorrhinum, Morbillinum and Tuberculinum, with their clear connection to specific named conditions, should have been used to describe the new remedies.

However, once the true nature of the body's vital (in the homeopathic sense) reaction was realised, a different relationship became apparent. The appearance of NLFB was neither the cause of, nor caused by, disease: the disease was present before the manifestation of the bacilli and that manifestation was in fact caused by a healing, rather than a disease driven, process. They were not products of disease processes as were discharges and effusions, but the products of a healing reaction.

The point to appreciate is that, in spite of the name, the bowel nosodes are not similar agents to other nosodes, and do not act in the same way. Other nosodes act on a disease situation, either as part of treatment in the acute illness, or to address the energetic memory imprint of that illness, or to correct imbalances in the 'soil' of potential sufferers. In contrast the bowel nosodes, with their source material being the result of a healing reaction within the body, act at the curative end of the 'dis-ease' spectrum and augment that curative action.

The animal connection

One of the constant queries of veterinary homeopathy in relation to all remedies is, since the basis of the provings and the bulk of the research is human orientated, whether it is valid to transfer the findings of such to the clinical situations that are encountered in animals. In the main, clinical experience indicates that there is a high degree of compatibility. However, most species of animals have, to varying degrees, a different digestive physiology to humans, especially in the case of the ruminant digestions of cattle, sheep and goats. Carnivore digestion is the closest to that of the human, and the digestive processes of horses, pigs, rabbits and guinea pigs fall somewhere between the two extremes. Hence in relation to the bowel nosodes the general question attains a particular relevance. Little work has been done in this regard, and such as there has been was linked to dogs and cats, the two species whose digestion is in many ways most similar to that of humans. General clinical experience, however, would indicate that across all the domestic mammalian species the clinical applications of the bowel nosodes as defined in humans are valid, which would be further indication that the essence of the reaction is systemic and fundamental rather than solely enteric. In addition, the confluence of the bacteriology in the large bowel that is seen across the species (see Chapter 3) would support the clinical findings. The remedies are found also to be clinically effective in birds. No data is available at present in relation to reptiles or fish.

In 1936 John Paterson reported on the clinical and bacteriological results of twelve thousand cases and indicated that NLFB were found in around twenty-five percent of those cases. In 1990 the author began taking faecal swabs from suitable animal cases that presented randomly at his surgery, and representing the range of conditions normally seen in practice. Suitable was defined as a new case that had not received any medication for any reason in the previous six months. The culturing and bacterial identification was carried out by a commercial laboratory following the method laid down by Paterson (1936, 1949) and using the bacterial classification of Alexander (1988). Over two and a half years faecal swabs were obtained from one hundred and seventy-four dogs and fifty-four cats. The results are given below:

The expression of the percentages to two decimal places may seem somewhat pedantic, especially in view of the considerably smaller number of animal specimens. However, that is how it was expressed in the original human work, and this has hence been reproduced.

[It should be noted that in the original publication of the work on animals (Saxton 1994), there was unfortunately a misinterpretation of the results leading to some false conclusions, particularly with regard to Faecalis. Readers of the original work should therefore ignore the quoted figures and the comments arising from them. The figures given above are correct.]

Representation of the other groups of NLFB was not found in the samples.

As stated above, the two species involved are those whose digestive physiology is closest to humans – in fact, some dogs are fed a human diet! Cats require a generally higher protein intake than either humans or canines and also lack the ability to synthesis the full range of amino acids that other species can. The majority of the animals included were being fed on commercial foods, the work being done before the increase in the use of raw diets that has occurred in recent years.

NLFB Group	J. Paterson %	Dogs %	Cats %
Morgan Bach	14.82	14.46	15.27
B. Proteus	3.73	2.87	1.85
B. Dysentery	1.77	0.00	0.00
B. Gaertner	1.27	0.00	0.00
B. Faecalis	0.86	0.91	0.67
B. No 7	0.82	1.15	0.00
B. Mutabile	0.46	1.72	0.00
Sycotic Co	0.32	0.57	1.85
	24.05	21.68	19.64

It is, of course, impossible to draw any firm conclusions from the above figures, but the comparison is interesting. Also of interest is the fact that forty percent of the cats yielding NLFB subsequently tested positive for Feline Leukaemia (Saxton 1994).

The management and financial constraints around the food producing species mean that true chronic disease is rarely if ever treated. An additional block to research in that direction is the fact that nowadays antibiotics are fed routinely to the animals as growth promoters or other performance enhancers.

3

BOWEL FLORA, IMMUNE FUNCTION AND HEALTH

Bowel function in relation to health

It is important to bear in mind that the function of the bowel is so much more than the mere processing of dietary intake and the resulting necessity elimination of the waste product of digestion (Hill D R 2010). The lining of the bowel is a direct extension of the skin and hence in a sense represents an external surface of the body, and thus like the skin the bowels have a major immune function. This function is manifest at the local level in the tissues of the intestinal mucosa of the lower bowel, and the efficiency with which this part of the immune system functions is intimately linked to the composition and balance of the bowel flora. However, because immune system is concerned with the health of the whole body, any impairment of function in one part can lead to the function of other areas being compromised. Hence alterations which are induced in the balance of the bowel flora can lead to upsets in the intestinal immunity which result in the appearance of symptoms elsewhere in the body. Similarly challenges to other parts of the immune system may be reflected in the intestinal mucosa, which in turn lead to changes in the bowel flora.

In health there is a balanced symbiotic relationship between the bowel flora and the rest of the body, often described by the term *eubiosis*. In In omnivores such as man, the carnivores and birds, all of which have a digestive system based on enzyme activity, the environment of the stomach and small intestine is not conducive to extensive bacterial development and action, and the relatively small numbers of mainly gram positive aerobic bacteria found in the anterior parts of the alimentary system remain essentially stable. The large intestine provides the environment in which bacteria can thrive and it is there that the balance changes and becomes a large population of predominantly gram negative and anaerobic bacteria of an essentially putrefactive or proteolytic nature. In contrast herbivores of both the single and multi-stomached varieties show significant activity of both anaerobic bacteria and protozoa in the anterior parts of the digestive system, largely for cellulose breakdown and carbohydrate digestion. However, in the large bowel there are corresponding changes to those seen in the omnivorous, carnivorous and avian species resulting in a similar range of bacterial activity in all (Dukes 1955). If for any reason the balanced state in any species is disturbed, this is described as a state of *dysbiosis*. Such a state may become established as a result of direct abuse to the alimentary system. These may arise as the result of dietary factors or the extended use of oral medication: prolonged or repeated courses of antibiotics or steroids will adversely affect the bowel flora, as will age. Systemic clinical conditions may provide a double hit on the bowel flora from both the primary condition and the medication that is used in its treatment. Over enthusiastic worming can contribute to a dysbiosis as can excessive purgation arising either as a result of sever detoxification regimes or as a prerequisite of investigative or clinical intervention such as colonoscopy or bowel surgery. Surgery of any sort with the necessary adjunct of anaesthesia has the potential for a major derangement of systemic function which can result in an upset to the balance of the bacterial flora of the lower part of the alimentary system. Other challenges and events which have an influence on other parts of the body, such as direct trauma or infection, will also influence the bowel flora. The physical symptom of diarrhoea mayor may not be present, although conditions involving prolonged diarrhoea have a greater potential to cause upsets. Constipation can also influence the bowel flora primarily as a result of the decreased peristalsis involved. However, It is not only frank physical events that can affect the bowels but mental factors such as stress or grief may be sufficient to impinge on the bowel's floral balance and create a dysbiosis. Another important cause is suppression of the body's normal response to disease or the medical suppression of a normal body function as with chemical contraception or Hormone Replacement Therapy. (In the author's opinion the routine surgical neutering of domestic animals when young (pre-puberty) does not produce the same effect since the whole potential function is, in effect, removed along with the reproductive organs. Problems may however arise if all or part of the ovaries are retained or when the procedure is carried out on sexually mature animals).

Whatever the cause, once established the disbiotic state in the bowels is capable of producing a systemic state of dis-ease, which may or may not result in a clinically recognised condition, or it may constitute an obstacle to cure in relation to any syndrome which is associated with it, no matter where in the body that syndrome's primary manifestation may be. Hence there is often a connection to the 'Never Well Since' aetiology what is utilised in homeopathic proscribing.

The exact bacterial make-up of the dysbiosis created in an individual case will be governed by the body's response to that particular challenge. That will first of all be influenced by the predominant miasmatic pattern of the individual patient. In addition there is the view that each and every challenge, of whatever sort, contains is own individual balance of the fundamental forces of creation, destruction and control that are found in nature (Saxton 2006). It is these same forces that underlie the basic misms and hence the exact response of an individual to a particular challenge will be the result of the interaction between the forces present in both body and challenge. This means that the bowel nosode that is indicated in a particular case will reflect the underlying miasmatic aspects of the whole situation. Similarly the balance of the associated remedies of each bowel nosode will reflect the underlying miasmatic pattern of the respective bowel nosode and the symptom picture linked to it.

In chronic disease various types of bacteria have been found with a weak ability to ferment lactose, and a tendency to move temporarily into a non-lactose fermenting state (Paterson 1949). In the case of the cocci associated with Sycotic Co the link is via their gram negative nature in primary culture (Paterson 1933). The administration of a well selected remedy, or where appropriate the indicated bowel nosode, stimulates the intestinal mucosa, as a part of the whole immune system, thereby triggering changes in the bacteria from lactose fermenting to non-lactose fermenting and these new forms then appear in the faeces as part of the elimination process. This change facilitates the return to the eubotic state, with a corresponding improvement in the health of the patient. It is this underlying recreation of a normal balanced bowel flora that ensures the maintainance of good health after the disappearance of the NLFB from the stool.

Bowel nosodes, pre- and pro-biotics and diet

The point that is often raised in criticism of the bowel nosodes is that changes in the bowel flora are easily achievable by means of diet alone. It is true that diet can have a marked effect on the intestinal flora. The widespread interest in and use of both pre and probiotics, established in the public mind as the contrast between 'good' and 'bad' bacteria, is based on that one fact. Probiotics have been defined as 'a live microbial feed supplement that beneficially affects the host animal by improving the intestinal microbial balance' (Fuller 1989). Prebiotics are complex hydrocarbons designed to enhance the effects of probiotics by providing optimal nutrition for the appropriate desired bacteria at the expense of other less desirable microbes. The use of these dietary agents derives from the approach that a healthy bowel will result in a healthy body. Whilst there is an acknowledgement that the gastrointestinal tract is involved in the whole immune function of the body, the emphasis is on the maintenance of the correct bowel flora as a major means of boosting the immune function, and the clinical indications for the use of probiotics are aimed essentially at creating such a normal bowel flora. In contrast homeopathy views the alimentary system and its mucus surfaces as an integral part of the overall immune system, just as all mucus surfaces of the body that are continuous with the skin (mouth, nose etc) have an important immune function. It has been shown (Chapter 2) that the NLFB which are the source material of the bowel nosodes are the result of a curative response by the whole body to a correct treatment and thus the resulting healthy bowel flora is the consequence of the development of a healthy body. It is the immune system rather than the bowels which provides the mechanism through which health is achieved and maintained.

Pre- and probiotics have been used have been used in a range of clinical conditions. Occasionally prebiotics may be used alone to selectively encourage the growth of particular bacteria that are already present in small numbers, thus favourably altering the balance of the bowel flora. More often probiotics, with or without prebiotics, are introduced in order to directly alter the flora, which may lead to the elimination of any undesirably organisms in the bowels. The author has on one occasion used probiotics successfully to clear an infestation of giardia (Giardia lamblia) in a dog where other treatments had failed.

Another technique employed for the introduction of new microbial material into the bowels is that of the faecal transplant (also called either faecal implant or trans-poo-sion), where faecal material from a donor is introduced directly into the bowel of the patient. The technique has grown in popularity in recent years and has been used successfully in conditions such as C. difficile infection and ulcerative colitis (Moaryyedi P 2017: Paramsothy 2018). Success often requires more than one implant and there is some anecdotal evidence to suggest that the results are improved if the donor has a blood relationship with the recipient.

Work at Yale (Rettiger & Cheplin 1921) demonstrated that:

(a) B Acidophilus given in whey broth cultures in sufficient amounts (300mls) can alter the bowel flora by suppressing or supplanting other organisms.

(b) Lactose when given in sufficient quantities (300–500 gms daily) can also change the bowel flora with the appearance and preponderance of B Acidophilus.

(c) By combining the administration of B Acidophilus with lactose comparatively small amounts were required to maintain the change in the bowel flora (150 gms lactose and 150 mls whey broth).

The first point to note is that all the changes observed were in response to the administration of local external agents. In addition it was found that the simple character of the new flora persists only as long as one diet or other preparation is continued, but reverts gradually to what was the normal or usual mixed type within five or six days after a return to the pre trail diet. Other attempts over a number of years to alter the bowel flora permanently by dietary means have met with various degrees of success but all have suffered from the same problem of reversion once the effective diet was removed (Paterson 1949). More recent work on probiotics in humans (Bouhnik 1992) and horses (Medina 2002) has confirmed the intrinsically transient nature of the effect. Also, clinical experience shows that treatment of gut dysbiosis solely by the addition of B Acidophilus to the diet produces at best only a temporary improvement that regresses to the original state when the supplement is discontinued. This temporary nature of such externally induced bowel changes is the basis for the routine use of pro-biotics as diet supplements, either as pure probiotics or as additions to various foods. However, the diet supplements of 'good bacteria' commonly available usually contain only one strain of Lactobacillus, which may or may not be appropriate to a particular situation.

This transient phenomenon is due to the fact that dietary additions have an influence only on the entirely free living portion of the bowel flora, without affecting in any way the more fixed portion that is closely associated with the surface of the alimentary mucosa (Medina 2002: Desrochers 2005: Malcolm 2007). These closely adhered bacteria have what could be considered to be a symbiotic relationship with the functioning of the immune system that provides the mechanism whereby eubiosis is maintained. When disease is present it is necessary to correct the underlying disturbance in the tissues of the alimentary mucosa by internal means if genuine progress towards cure is to be made (Asher 2006).

Where a bowel nosode is indicated the NLFB are produced as the result of an internal stimulation, of short duration, of the whole body system by the administration of a potentised remedy, and as has been demonstrated previously (Chapter 2) there is no intrinsic difference between a remedy and the particular bowel nosode associated with it. Such stimulation cannot in any way be described as a food supplement or diet adjustment. Nor is the effect very quickly apparent, usually requiring somewhere between the ten and fourteen days of a genuine immune response (cf vaccination). In addition once the NLFB have appeared they will persist for periods of weeks or months, without further stimulation, before gradually waning and finally disappearing. Cases of NLFB persisting for up to fourteen months have been recorded and during that time changes in the diet were found to have no further effect on the bowel flora (Paterson 1949). It was also found to be impossible, once the NLFB had appeared, to alter further the bowel flora by the administration of additional homeopathic remedies (Paterson 1933: but see the case on page 000)

The best that can be expected from short term diet changes or the administration of probiotics is a purely externally induced, temporary and essentially passive reaction in the body, which may be sufficient in situations where a short term solution is all that is required. In chronic cases however the only way the required changes can be maintained is by the continued application of the external stimulation. In contrast potentised remedies induce an internal active and permanent response which does not require further regular stimulation. In the discussion following the presentation of his paper *The Potentised Drug and its Action on the Bowel Flora* (1936) John Paterson was asked if he recommended a standardised diet for his patients. His answer was 'no' as 'if a patient were fed on certain foods the environment in the bowel was altered but not the person. Homeopathic remedies would alter the individual and indirectly the flora of the bowel.'

4

THE CLINICAL APPLICATIONS

General considerations

Although there are some indications for the bowel nosodes in the genuinely acute situation, their overwhelming usefulness is in the treatment of chronic disease. Some apparently acute episodes will, of course, be periodic acute manifestations of an underlying chronic condition. John Paterson said that 'one should not expect too much of the bowel nosodes' (1949) but others feel that this is to underestimate their usefulness (Brown 1967; Somper 2002). As indicated previously, the scope for their use extends across both man and the domestic animals, and there is no reason to suppose that their use would not be applicable in wild species also. The author has on occasion used them with success in captive parrots. Over the years the taking of a faecal swab has been both the main research tool of the work and an integral part of the remedy selection process. Elizabeth Paterson (1960) based all three hundred and thirty of her recorded cases on the results of a swab.

However, although the taking of faecal swabs is still a legitimate technique, in practice a suitable unadulterated bowel flora, especially without the influence of antibiotics, on which to base its use is becoming increasingly rare. Hence, while it is still a possible approach, it is unlikely to find much application in the present medical climate. In addition, although the required laboratory procedures are not too demanding, they are unlikely to form part of a modern laboratory's standard range. The method is included below as a means of demonstrating the whole concept. The reader is referred to the case at the end of this chapter (page 00) for the clinical context of its use.

The other methods of use outlined in this chapter are based on current clinical experience and interpretation of the unique relationships of the bowel nosodes discussed in Chapter 2. It should be noted that John Paterson was always insistent that when there was a clear indication for a particular remedy in a case, then that remedy should always be used in preference to the bowel nosode. He also cautioned when using the nosodes to '. . . remember that they are deep acting remedies and cover the totality of symptoms from the highest level, the 'mentals' to the lowest level of 'gross pathology' and that they also cover the life history of the patient from earliest childhood to adult life or old age'.

The faecal swab

The interpretation of the swab result would have depended on an assessment of the effect that the illness was having on the patient, and it was appropriate also to remember the positive and negative phases of chronic disease as described by Wheeler and Bach (Chapter 1).

There are various results that may be obtained from the culture of a swab, and each will indicate a different course of action.

(i) *A particular group of NLFB present at over 50%*

Do not give the bowel nosode associated with the NLFB at this stage. This result indicates a positive phase of the disease cycle and clinically the patient may well appear to be in reasonable health at this time. This situation is most likely to be encountered in an old case that has received previous homeopathic treatment with a degree of success. As the presence of large numbers of NLFB indicates that there is some genuine healing reaction occurring, the body's own defences are obviously controlling the 'dis-ease' to a reasonable extent, but yet are not able to proceed to a final cure on their own. Giving the bowel nosode at this time is contra-indicated, and John Paterson (1949) cites his experience of this causing a reversal of the healing process, driving the patient back into the negative phase of the disease and producing a depression of the body's vitality. What is required at this stage is some gentle augmentation of that existing healing process. This may be achieved by either giving a specifically indicated remedy from the appropriate list of associated remedies or, if there is no clear choice, using a leading remedy from the list. If there is more than one such remedy, select the most indicated even though the symptom picture is incomplete. Low to moderate potency should be employed.

(ii) *A particular group of NLFB present at less that 30%*

This represents a negative phase of the disease, where the disease is in the ascendancy over the healing reaction. The presence of the NLFB indicates that there is some healing action but it is being swamped by the illness. Here the patient will present as being clinically worse than in the situation above.

This is an indication for the bowel nosode as identified by the NLFB group. The healing reaction requires stimulation on a deep level. As has been shown (Chapter 2), the bowel nosode that has been identified will be homeopathic for the disease, and will hence be an appropriate remedy selection. The potency used should be in the moderate range.

(iii) *A group of NLFB identified at a level of between 30–50%*

From this single result it is impossible to tell if the disease is moving towards either a negative or positive phase. The recent history of the patient may give some indication, but even that can be unclear. It may be that the patient is remaining in a state of uneasy balance with no significant changes in health either way. This uncertain state requires a gentle rather than a vigorous stimulation, and hence the potency given should be low. There are two choices in this situation. The first is to use the remedy in the associated list that is the best match, even though it may not be a good match. The alternative is to give the appropriate bowel nosode.

(iv) *Some NLFB found but identification with a specific group is not possible*

In this situation the percentage of NLFB found will be low. It represents a very weak healing reaction, and one that therefore needs stimulating. That lack of reaction may, of course, be linked to a low vitality on the part of the patient. A low potency is all that is indicated. Experience has shown that the two remedies that are most appropriate in this situation are Merc Sol. and Tuberculinum. The ideal choice between the two depends on being able to identify any matching symptoms that are present although John Paterson regarded Merc Sol. as the more important of the two remedies in this regard (1948). Hence in the absence of any guiding symptoms the Mercury should be used. The result is often to give a boost to the patient's system and as a consequence produce a clarification of the bacteriological picture. This, of course, implies a second swab, usually some two to three weeks later.

Why it should be these two remedies that are indicated is unclear. It may be that, as they both have a broad action, enough of a 'similar' is given to act as a healing stimulus. Aiming, as it were, for such a broad action implies a low potency whatever the vitality of the patient may be.

(v) *A negative result*

The picture here is similar to that described above and the required action is the same.

Other methods of using the bowel nosodes

In addition to the detailed symptoms found in the remedy schemas of each of the bowel nosodes, each one also has key themes that, in a number of prescribing situations, can be used to direct the practitioner. These are discussed in more depth as those situations are dealt with, and in the individual chapters. The themes are listed in outline later in this chapter and a knowledge of them can aid greatly in utilising the nosodes. (The term 'keynotes 'will often be found used in connection with the broad characteristics of the individual bowel nosodes. However, as the nuances of the individual nosodes are better understood, the term 'themes' appears to be more appropriate, as the characteristics described are more analogous to the themes being identified in the various kingdoms by modern workers such as Massimo Mangialavori, Sankaran and Scholten.) As homeopathy does not make the distinction between mind and body that is found in orthodox western medicine, it should be remembered that the themes of the individual nosodes apply equally at both the mental and physical levels.

The following are the methods in which the bowel nosodes may be incorporated into case management. It will be noted that most of these are concerned with chronic conditions and obstacles to progress in a case.

(i)   *As remedies in their own right*

All of the bowel nosodes have their own remedy picture and, if that fits the presenting symptoms in a case, they may be prescribed in exactly the same way as any other remedy. Where there are acute indications for the nosodes, it is as such individual remedies that they are used. Some of the nosodes lend themselves to this usage more than others. John Paterson considered that Proteus and Sycotic Co. were the two of most value in this regard but Morgan Bach, Dysentery Co. and Mutabile (Brown 1989; Somper 1988) have also been shown to have acute indications. Details of each will be found in the relevant chapters. The characteristic theme is often a major factor in the selection of one of the nosodes to be used in this individual way. It must also be stated again that what appears at first sight to be an acute condition may in fact be an acute manifestation of an underlying chronic state, and the use of a bowel nosode in such circumstances may open a case completely and address its deepest levels.

(ii) *To clear a symptom picture*

In this situation the nosode may be used in one of two ways. The first is to clear the effects of previous conventional medication from the system, in the same way as other remedies such as Nux Vomica or

Sulphur are used. There are slight differences between the indications for these two remedies in this regard, with Sulphur being used when there has been an overuse of one particular medication whilst Nux Vomica is selected when it is desired to clear the effects of multiple medications. Similarly the bowel nosodes may be used with two slightly different indications. The use of a particular nosode is indicated when there has been the use of one specific type of medication, for example Gaertner Bach following antibiotics. If there have been a number of medications employed previously, then it is usually more efficacious to select the bowel nosode on the basis of the relevance of its theme to the basic condition. The use of either of these techniques will result in the appearance of a symptom picture that is more truly representative of the underlying problem, thus allowing a more accurate remedy selection to be made.

If, in spite of a full case-taking, it proves impossible to differentiate clearly between a number of remedies, then another form of using a bowel nosode to clear the situation can be employed. If the choice of potential remedies lies between members of the same associated remedy list, then the bowel nosode connected to that list should be administered. If either the choice of remedies is widely based and cuts across more than one list, or the available symptoms are so generalised or unclear so as to make accurate selection impossible, then the use of a bowel nosode selected on its theme is a helpful way forward. With either of these approaches, a clearer picture on which to prescribe should emerge.

It should also be remembered that the bowel nosodes as a group have strong connections to the miasms and hence consideration of any miasmatic pattern discernable in a case can provide an additional clue to the selection of an appropriate nosode.

Although not widely used nowadays, an alternative approach in those cases where there is no definite remedy group indicated was suggested by John Paterson (1953). This was to use the mixture Poly Bowel (Bach) (see Chapter 1) to start the case. His rationale for this was that, as Morgan Bach was in fact a mixture of two individual nosodes (see Chapter 4), and as it was often used because it was impossible to differentiate the indications of the two individual nosodes in a case, he could see no theoretical obstacle to combining a greater number of all the bowel nosodes in one preparation if the vagueness of the presenting picture warranted it. Conversely, others have warned against the practice of mixing the nosodes in a case (Agrawal 1995), on the grounds that it is casting the net too wide to produce the desired effect. However, it must be remembered that the desired effect in these cases is merely to change and clarify a symptom picture, not to make a specific and individual prescription. Also, in such cases, the degree of dysbiosis present may be so great as to verge on being an obstacle to cure, and this may be helped by the broader spectrum approach. The author's view is that Poly Bowel does have a role where a more specific indication cannot be identified, although it should never be considered for routine use.

(iii) *When a well selected remedy fails to act or has only a short duration*
The first requirement here is to check that in fact the remedy is well selected, which will mean returning to the case and reassessing it. If the remedy remains indicated, and other reasons for its failing to act, such as damage to the remedy, incorrect potency or failure of owner/patient compliance are eliminated, then the administration of the appropriate bowel nosode is indicated. This may or may not produce an apparent effect. If it does, then the case is taken forward in accordance with normal second prescription protocols. If there is no obvious effect, then a return to the originally selected remedy will often produce the desired effect.

In some cases where the correct remedy has been administered, it may be found that its action is of short duration only, after which the clinical picture reverts to its initial form. The recognised response to this event is to administer the same remedy again, but at a different potency. The potency change is usually upwards. If the same pattern of temporary improvement is seen again, then the use of the associated bowel nosode will often break through the block. The administration of the nosode may produce progress of itself or, as above, there may be little apparent effect. In the latter instance a return to the selected remedy is the way forward, usually at the original potency employed. A similar indication for the nosode is where there has been a definite but limited response to the initial remedy, and although that is maintained no further progress can be achieved with that remedy in any potency, even though it still remains indicated. The use of the nosode as described above is a way forward.

A variation of this stimulus action of the bowel nosodes on associated remedies has been employed by some practitioners (Somper 2002). Having taken the case and selected a remedy, the bowel nosode associated with it is administered prior to the giving the remedy, which is then given closely following the nosode. The two courses may be given consecutively. The rationale is that the nosode either directly augments the action of a remedy that was going to have an effect anyway, or by correcting the dysbiosis present it prevents the blocks described above from developing, and hence enables the remedy to have its effect immediately. The author has used the technique on occasion and the subsequent responses have been excellent. The objection can be raised that this approach risks giving the nosode in a positive phase of the disease, but careful selection and assessment of the case should avoid that.

It has also been noted as a clinical fact that if the interval between the administration of the bowel nosode and the repeat of the previously 'blocked' remedy is too great, then the beneficial effect is decreased and in many cases finally lost. The exact critical interval will vary depending on the individual case, but the aim should be always to keep the interval to the minimum.

(iv) *Using an indicated remedy and its associated bowel nosode together*
This is a form of the accepted treatment protocol of using a local remedy together with a constitutional prescription. In this instance it is the bowel nosode that fulfils the role of the constitutional remedy, being essentially a deep-acting remedy, as discussed previously. The remedy is selected primarily on the more local aspects of the case, although mental and/or general symptoms should be taken account of wherever possible. The bowel nosode associated with that remedy is then used. Following the usual potency guide in this approach, the bowel nosode is given in the higher potency with the locally prescribed remedy administered in the lower.

(v) *To overcome great sensitivity to a well selected remedy*
Problems occur occasionally when a particular patient has an unusual sensitivity to a well-selected remedy. In many cases this implies that it has been very well selected and hence the desirability of continuing with it. (The other aspect of this is, of course, that the better the selection the less need there will be for repeat doses.) In other instances there may be considerations of a patient or animal welfare nature, with other symptoms from the remedy picture, such as pain, appearing albeit temporarily, that are deemed unacceptable and hence require treatment. An associated bowel nosode should be considered in these cases.

(vi) *To clear persistent symptoms or a general failure to thrive after acute illness*
An aetiology of 'Never Well Since' (NWS) is itself a strong indication for the use of a bowel nosode. In these cases the remedy that was

correctly chosen based on the symptoms of the presenting acute disease has failed to address the chronic underlying aspects of the 'disease'. The bowel nosode selected should be the one most strongly associated with the remedy that has produced the improvement in the acute phase of the illness.

Key themes of the bowel nosodes

The key themes of the bowel nosodes are as follows:

Morgan Bach
Congestion

Dysentery Co.
Anticipatory anxiety, nervous tension

Proteus
Suddenness, nervous system involvement

Sycotic Co.
Irritability

Gaertner Bach
Malnutrition, emaciation

Bacillus No. 7
Mental and physical fatigue

Bacillus No. 10
Fluorine (lack of restraint, destructive pushing of boundaries)

Mutabile
Changeability

Faecalis
Mental dichotomy (JS – see below)

Coccal Co.
Infection and septic states

The theme of Gaertner Bach is generally quoted as malnutrition but emaciation should also be included in the picture (see Chapter 8)

The description linked to Faecalis requires explanation, as in most lists of the themes this is just stated as 'Sepia'. The idea of 'mental dichotomy' (or 'duality') is the author's own, based on the two remedies that have been identified as being associated. Anacardium has the classic description of 'an angel on one shoulder and a devil on the other', while Sepia has the constant tug between duty and desire. Many remedies, of course, have contrasting mental symptoms, such as Graphites whose intellectual and emotional aspects have been compared by Coulter (1998). However, it is the marked degree of conflict between mental traits within a personality when manifest in a remedy that justifies the 'duality' description. Both Anacardium and Sepia have this conflict and it may be that other remedies with a similar feature could be considered for inclusion under Faecalis. Thuja and Sulphur have both been suggested as being linked (Elliott 1996 – see Chapter 10) Thuja's potential mental detachment and unworldliness may be an indication of its duality and the forked urine stream found in its picture is a physical aspect of the state. Carcinosin and Lachesis are two other possible remedies to be included.

Often, only Calc Fluor. is quoted in the associated remedy list for Bacillus No. 10 and from that it is more difficult to give a clear generalised theme to this nosode as a basis for prescribing. However, other remedies, notably the predominantly sycotic Thuja and Nat Sulph. have been mentioned in this context and this will alter the perception of the nosode. The 'lack of restraint' mentioned above could apply as much to the excessive creation of tissue seen typically in the sycotic miasm as to the destructive loss of boundaries seen in fluorine and the syphilitic miasm. (See Chapter 10 for further discussion of this point.)

Dosage considerations

The general recommendation for the use of the bowel nosodes is that they should be used in a 30c potency and not be repeated within three months. Not repeating within three months was a particularly strong recommendation of both Drs John and Elizabeth Paterson. In addition to not repeating the bowel nosodes too frequently, only short courses should be employed in most cases where they are used. Often only a single dose is required, or the pattern of three doses in twenty-four hours with twelve hours between doses (the 'single divided dose'). In animals a regime of night and morning for up to four days is often employed. The question of whether, due to the shorter life expectancy of the animal species, the three month rule should be adjusted accordingly is the cause of some debate within the veterinary homeopathic community. Certainly on many occasions the author has broken the 'three month rule' without disastrous results, and veterinary experience generally indicates much greater flexibility over both frequency and potency than has been traditionally recommended in the human medical world (Elliott 1993). The author will never hesitate to change the prescription of a bowel nosode at any time interval provided the progress of the case indicates such a move. Equally, if a bowel nosode is being used as an acute remedy, then the normal rules of acute prescribing are applied.

Most of the potency recommendations of John Paterson in his papers envisage the use of the nosodes without the backup of a laboratory, which is the normal situation today. Brown (1989) tells of his experience of observing the Patersons at work over many years, and comments on the narrow range of potencies that they used generally, concentrating largely on the lower end of the scale, from 3x up to 30c. Apparently a 200c was avoided at all costs, and a 1M was considered a very high potency. John Paterson confirms this view in his 1953 paper, recommending reserving higher potencies for acute disease. However, in his 1949 address in Lyon, he speaks of using the nosodes at 1M or higher where there are strong mental symptoms. At the other end of the scale he recommends 6c where there is any advanced pathology, including malignancy, and speaks of a daily dose over a period 'determined by clinical observation'. When using a remedy and a bowel nosode together, he selected the accompanying remedy on the broadest possible range of symptoms and, if sure of his choice, would give three times daily for up to a month (Brown 1989). The objective was not to select a purely local remedy but rather one with as wide a coverage of the case as possible, and to use it to support and augment the action of the nosode. Also in the Lyon lecture (1949) he recommends the use of 6c in cases that have received potentised remedies within one month prior to administering a nosode, pointing out that any remedy that has had a degree of success may well have altered the bowel flora from its original disease state. Mention is also made of the value of the 30c potency in those cases where there is a tendency within a case to acute episodes within a framework of chronic disease. However, Sankaran P (1984) is more tolerant of the higher potencies generally and Kennedy also speaks of their use. The author is now making increasing use of potency chords, most commonly over the range of 6c, 30c and 200c, and very occasionally from 30c to 1m. Their mode of action appears ideally suited to the deep action of the bowel nosodes. (A fuller discussion of potency chords will be found in the Appendix.)

A tendency to diarrhoea has been reported in cats following the use of bowel nosodes (von Schreiber 2008). This should be remembered in the context of dosage, from the point of view of both potency and frequency of administration.

It is clear that the bowel nosodes are not immune to differences of opinion over potency any more than other areas of homeopathic prescribing. Many of the recommendations for their use follow widely accepted rules, but in addition it is as well to remember two things about them. Firstly, their very deep and long-acting nature and secondly, exactly where they fit into the healing processes of the body and how this can be utilised.

Case 4.1 (from Dr John Paterson)

Brown (1967) quotes a case treated by John Paterson in which he used a bowel nosode to clear the symptom picture initially and then relied on repeated faecal swabs at three to four-month intervals to guide him.

This case concerned a lady with a primary diagnosis of asthma who had received both conventional and homeopathic treatment prior to his involvement. In view of the previous medication the initial prescription was of Nux Vom. as a general cleansing remedy followed by the taking of a faecal swab. This indicated Morgan Bach as the remedy of choice, which was duly administered in a 30c. The resulting changes produced a symptom picture of Kali Carb. which was then given. Over time the symptom picture changed and it became clear that the case was in fact more complicated than it at first appeared, with symptoms of both bowel colic and urticaria entering the picture. Treatment through it all was directed by the particular NLFB produced at various stages pointing to particular bowel nosodes or groups of remedies. In view of the reasons already discussed, such an approach will not usually be a practical clinical option nowadays. During the course of the disease the NLFB picture moved through Morgan Bach, Mutabile and Sycotic Co.

Unfortunately, greater detail of the treatment was not reported, especially the time scale involved; nor was the final outcome, although the implication was that the case was cured. However, enough insight is there to give several points of interest. There was firstly the use of a bowel nosode to clear the symptom picture, with the subsequent use of a remedy indicated by the revealed symptoms. Secondly, the true, deep-seated nature of chronic disease is demonstrated together with the action of the bowel nosodes in reaching those depths. Allied to that is the changing pattern of the NLFB as each new layer was revealed. The miasmatic balance in a case can change as successful treatment moves it in the direction of cure

(Saxton 2006) such a pattern is seen here with the emergence of a sycotic aspect of the case (Mutabile and Sycotic Co.) when the presenting psoric (Morgan Bach) manifestation had been addressed. It would have been interesting to know whether there was a return to psora as the final stage of cure, but unfortunately that information was not provided.

5

THE MORGAN GROUP
Morgan Bach, Morgan Pure and Morgan Gaertner

General considerations

Morgan Bach represents the group of NLFB that were isolated initially by Dr Bach, and the whole group forms the basis of the nosode Morgan Bach (known also as Morgan Co.) which was the first bowel nosode to be isolated by Edward Bach and which is still widely used today, especially in the veterinary field where obtaining the full symptom picture can be more diffi-cult than in the human field. Subsequent work by Dr Paterson resulted in two distinct groups of bacteria being identified within that whole. The tech-nique of culturing for eighteen hours had produced the sugar reactions that distinguished the group as a whole. However, it was found that by continu-ing the incubation for the full seventy-two hours more generally used in laboratory investigations, differences in the fermentation reactions of some of the bacteria began to appear. Some retained their fermentation reactions unchanged after the longer incubation, and these were designated as the Morgan Pure group, since they remained true to their original form. Others, however, had produced reactions in the sugar dulcitol that had not been present after only eighteen hours, and those reactions had become similar to those seen at eighteen hours by the Gaertner Bach group of NLFB (Pater-son 1949). Accordingly, this group was called the Morgan Gaertner group.

Both these groups of NLFB have given rise to bowel nosodes, named Morgan Pure and Morgan Gaertner respectively, in addition to Morgan Bach which is the nosode prepared from the combined groups of NLFB. The Morgan group as a whole is the one most commonly identified in the clinical situation. John Paterson found that sixty percent of his positive results yielded the whole Morgan Bach group, whilst Elizabeth Paterson in her review of cases recorded Morgan Pure in fifty percent of the results with slightly over another twenty percent showing Morgan Gaertner. The

Morgan Bach group was also the most commonly identified in both Dr John's swab survey and the author's pilot replication study (see Chapter 2).

There are considerable overlaps in the materia medica of Morgan Pure and Morgan Gaertner, but there are also some differences. Although there are occasions where it is appropriate to utilise the more specific match of either Morgan Pure or Morgan Gaertner, in many clinical situations it is the combined nosode that is used. As discussed in Chapter 3, this is because in many cases it is impossible to ascertain the particular symptoms needed to differentiate between the two nosodes. Hence it is appropriate to consider the broad picture of the nosodes representing the group as one under the heading of 'Morgan Bach' and then to consider the differences of the two sub groups. The key theme of the nosodes is *congestion* and it runs through the materia medica of all three. The main action is on the skin and mucous membranes, especially of the alimentary tract, including the liver. Sulphur and carbon are the two most consistent elements among the associated remedies, and John Paterson (1953a) linked the redness seen in the picture to the influence of sulphur whereas the carbon produces a more static and passive state.

One of the differences between the two sub-groups appears in connection with the alimentary and skin symptoms (Paterson 1949c). Morgan Pure is linked to skin eruptions and/or liver disturbances of a chronic nature; and whilst Morgan Gaertner also has a major effect on the liver, it is indicated more when there is, or has been, an acute inflammatory attack involving the liver and gall bladder. Morgan Pure has been linked to painful conditions triggered by the presence of gallstones. Morgan Gaertner has similar connections to renal colic and calculi, especially where the pain first occurs on the left side, although the calculi are often found in both kidneys. The leading remedy of the Morgan Gaertner group is Lycopodium and the other remedies often indicated in liver conditions, such as Chelidonium and Taraxacum, are represented also. Lycopodium has the strong modality of < 4–8pm, which is also a modality of the nosode Morgan Gaertner. Similarly the 11am 'sinking empty feeling > eating' seen in Sulphur is also found in the Morgan Pure picture.

Although not quite a specific, the use of Morgan Bach in tracheobronchitis (kennel cough in the dog) is strongly indicated. It use in bronchopneumonia may be indicated, and most cases of eczema in children will benefit from the nosode at some stage of their treatment (Paterson 1949). Skin conditions that will benefit are generally < heat. Morgan Bach has also been recommended for use in malignant states in the elderly (Paterson 1953). It is relevant also for conditions where there is a history of repeated inflammatory attacks.

The main miasmatic influences running through the nosode are those of psora and sycosis. Because of the connection with the skin, psora tends to be emphasised at the expense of sycosis, and this is a mistake. Although psora is undoubtedly the major of the two influences – and John Paterson considered that the nosode epitomised the psoric miasm (1953) – in fact sycosis makes a significant contribution to the symptom picture, and specific sycotic features, such as an aggravation from storms, will be seen. Of the two individual nosodes, Morgan Pure has the stronger connection to the psoric miasm.

Materia medica of Morgan group

Morgan Bach

On the general level the nosode is ameliorated by movement but aggravated by heat, especially that of the bed. There is also an aggravation at night.

The mental picture is one of general anxiety, introspection and depression extending to a desire to commit suicide by jumping; this is characteristic of the syphilitic miasm, emphasising the fact that all three miasms are always represented in every remedy (Saxton 2006). Concern for his/her general health is a feature; also fear of crowds and company, together with a dislike of being left alone. Nervous tension gives a restlessness and desire to be active. There is restless sleep or insomnia, but with a desire to sleep after eating.

The congestive theme is shown in the headaches that are accompanied by flushing of the face. They are generally worse for heat and thunder. It is a remedy for migraines, especially if occurring at regular intervals and accompanied by nausea. Excitement of any kind, but particularly travelling, may precipitate an attack. However, Agrawal (1995) does not consider it a major remedy in this regard. Vertigo caused by hypertension is seen. Non-purulent conjunctivitis is seen plus other inflammatory and cystic conditions of the eye and surrounding tissues, such as keratitis, iritis and blepharitis. Catarrhal conditions of the ear are found and the nosode has been mentioned as a major remedy in Ménière's disease.

Mention has been made of tracheobronchitis and bronchopneumonia as indications for the nosode, which is a reflection of the inflammatory and congestive processes that occur in the respiratory system. This may ultimately result in emphysema. Repetitive attacks of any respiratory condition, including asthma, may call for the remedy, especially those that occur in children and/or are manifest in the winter or spring. Copious nasal catarrh with thin clear or white discharge is seen. Inflammatory conditions of the throat can lead to choking, and burning sensations in the mouth are reported by patients, especially in the morning.

Congestion of the alimentary system leads to abdominal pain, especially in the upper or anterior abdomen. Gastric inflammation results in heartburn and a tendency to nausea, 'bilious attacks', recurrent indigestion with flatulence and a bitter taste in the mouth. The sense of taste may be lost. Ulceration of the anterior digestive system can finally occur, and idiopathic vomiting in cats may respond. Nausea linked to the menopause is a strong indication. There is a desire for butter and other fats, sweets and eggs, even though fats and eggs may aggravate any bowel conditions. There is a tendency towards constipation with dry stools although looseness may occur in the mornings, with urgency: the motion is foul smelling with some blood and mucus and is passed without straining. There is often a desire to pass a motion after food. Irritation around the anus without obvious cause is encountered, as are anal fistulae.

The cardiovascular system is involved with, at one extreme, hypertension and angina, whilst at the other extreme sluggish congestion leads to phlebitis, varicose veins, haemorrhoids and cyanosis of the extremities. The poor circulation in the extremities produces a predisposition to chilblains. There is discomfort around the heart, with nocturnal palpitations that are better for passing wind and movement.

The genital system is another major seat of action for Morgan Bach. Once more congestion features largely. Headaches linked to the function of the genital system, especially at the menopause, are often accompanied by ovarian pain and flushes. Other functional upsets produce both menorrhagia and metrorrhagia, whilst polyps and fibroids develop. Leucorrhoea may be either yellow to green or a definite brown, with a tendency to be corrosive. There is great irritation of the vagina and vulva.

The urinary system shows cystitis and frequency. During attacks the urine is strong-smelling and corrosive, giving burning pain on micturition. Enuresis is a feature.

The musculoskeletal system is involved with rheumatic and arthritic symptoms involving particularly the shoulders, arms, wrists, hands and knees. Pain may be experienced in the soles of the feet. Joints are swollen and painful, especially at night. General loss of power and stiffness in the limbs is accompanied by sensory nerve involvement giving tingling and numbness in the extremities. The grip of the hands is weakened and the sense of touch is reduced.

It is, however, with the skin that the nosode is most closely associated, and in this context it is Morgan Pure that contributes the majority of symptoms. All areas of the body may be affected, but behind the ears and the flexion aspect of the joints are worthy of special mention. Weeping eczema with crusts accompanied by great irritation and heat is seen. Two of the bacteria that form part of the nosode, Morganella Morganii and Proteus Mirabilis, are capable of synthesising histamine (Malcolm 2007) and this is reflected in the skin symptoms that arise. There is an almost irresistible urge to scratch, leading to bleeding in many instances. Animals will lick at their feet to the extent of producing swelling of the whole area. Equally, the skin may be dry and cracked with fissures but still irritant. In humans one pointer towards Morgan Bach is the presence of circinate lesions on the skin, although this is not seen to the same extent in animals. There is great thickening of the skin generally, and commonly of the heels, which are cracked and fissured. Warts are also present, often large and either flat or jagged. Skin conditions are usually worse for heat with sensitivity to the sun, washing and teething.

Morgan Pure

Traditionally associated remedies
Alumina, Baryta Carb, Calc Carb, Calc Sulph, Carbo Veg, Carbo Sulph, Digitalis Purp, Ferrum Carb, *Graphites*, Kali Carb, Mag Carb, *Medorrhinum*, Natrum Carb, Petroleum, *Psorinum*, Sepia Off, **Sulphur**, Tuberculinum Bov.

Within the general framework of the 'Morgan' group described above, Morgan Pure has its own additional individual features. As mentioned, it is specifically linked to skin and/or liver conditions of a chronic nature. It is a major remedy for eczema in young children. As well as the aggravation from heat seen through the whole group, Morgan Pure is aggravated by washing. It is also generally better for eating. The headaches of Morgan Pure are congestive and may be accompanied by the vomiting of mucus and bile. Migraine is frequently triggered by the onset of menstruation.

Mentally the type is introverted and unstable. Fears and anxieties, especially over health, may lead to thoughts of suicide. Nameless fears predominate and although there may be a great fear of particular diseases, such as cancer, there is often a general dread of just being ill. Inflammatory conditions of the mouth and throat produce dryness and redness of the mucosa. Ulcers and swelling of the tissues are seen, with salivation. Either dryness or catarrh may be found in the nasal region, together with sinusitis. and epistaxis. The respiratory system is particularly affected in the winter and spring, with bronchitis and bronchopneumonia tending to recur each year. There is a dry cough and shortness of breath with tightness in the chest, especially at night.

The congestion of the circulatory system produces a bluish tinge to the surface of the body in areas affected by varicose veins and phlebitis. In the urinary system there is painful cystitis with burning, but no blood. Glycosuria is present in the picture. Fibroids and ovarian pains are found in the genital system.

The skin is extremely irritant with great sensitivity to touch. There may be fissures and exudation or dry inflammation. Moist eczema occurs in children. Skin lesions may be linked to allergic responses, as in atopic dermatitis in the dog. Complete hair loss may be seen in humans, whilst in animals the coat is thin with areas of alopecia and constant hair loss over the whole body.

MORGAN PURE	
Mind	Introverted. Depression to point of suicide. Nameless fears especially of disease. Fear of crowds. Retarded development in young. Restlessness.
Head	Congestive headaches, migraine with nausea. Vertigo.
Face	Flushed face. Inflammatory conditions of eyes. Inflamed mucosa with dryness and mouth ulcers. Jaundice.
Abdomen	Pain in anterior areas. Heartburn. and nausea. Morning urgency for loose stools. Constipation. Gallstones.
Appetite	Desires fats, sweets and eggs. < fats and eggs.
Cardiovascular	Hypertension. Passive congestion.
Urogenital	Cystitis. Glycosuria. Ovarian pains. Fibroids. Corrosive leucorrhoea.
Respiratory	Bronchitis and pneumonia especially in spring. Asthma.
Musculoskeletal	Rheumatism and arthritis. Swollen painful joints.
Sleep	Poor. Restless. Desire to sleep after eating.
Skin	Great irritation. Weeping eczema. Redness. Hair loss.
Modalities & General	< heat, bathing, night, thunder > movement, eating. Sensitive to antibiotics.

Morgan Gaertner

Traditionally associated remedies
Chelidonium Maj, Chenopodium Ant, Helleborus Niger, Hepar Sulph, *Lachesis Muta*, **Lycopodium Clav**, Merc Sulph, Sanguinaria Can, Taraxacum Off.

Morgan Gaertner is linked to the liver and gall bladder, especially where acute inflammatory conditions are or have been present. It also has a strong association with the kidneys and renal calculi, and nephritis and pyelitis are seen. Kidney problems in cats are said to respond to the nosode, especially if there is an emotional element in the aetiology of the condition. It is generally worse for eating. The type is self-centred and can be self-pitying, with irritability and frank temper if crossed or contradicted. This shows especially in cats who will bite if crossed. There is a fear of company and yet, paradoxically, a fear of being alone. Tension can lead to nailbiting. Headaches are seen in which, although there may be a flushed face and a hot skin, the patient will often feel cold. The onset of headaches can be linked to genital function, particularly the menopause, and they are accompanied by ovarian pain and flushes. Migraine occurs just prior to the onset of menses. Against the general symptom of the nosode, headaches are relieved by eating. Premenstrual tension is a feature of the nosode. Sleep patterns are poor with unpleasant dreams, and eating produces tiredness. The nasal catarrh is associated with ulceration and bleeding. The mouth has generally a dirty appearance with thick saliva.

There is flatulence and distension of the abdomen with much borgorygmi that is often worse in the afternoon. The nosode is associated with more flatulence than any of the other bowel nosodes, and the patient is better for passage of the flatulence, which is usually foul-smelling, in either or both directions. The liver is tender and aggravated by palpation, especially in the region of the gall bladder. Jaundice is an indication. Both stomach and abdomen have feelings of fullness and distension. The tendency is towards constipation linked to weak bowel action, and even a normal motion may contain mucus. There is a desire for sweets, salt and hot food.

In the picture there is pain under the shoulderblades and the iliac fossae, mainly on the right but also on the left to some degree: in animals this may be severe enough to appear as lameness. In common with its leading remedy, Lycopodium, the nosode exhibits an idiopathic temperature difference between the feet, with the right feeling warmer to the touch than the left. In animals both front and/or hind legs may be affected and in humans there have been reports of the hands also being involved (Khan 2007).

Skin symptoms are present and can be triggered by contact with metal such as choke chains in dogs or jewellery in people. Anal fistulae, piles and prolapsed rectum are found. When hair loss occurs it is in discrete bunches rather than as a generalised loss. Pustules are seen.

MORGAN GAERTNER

Mind	Self-centred. Anxious. Short-tempered. Jealous. Fear of crowds, company and being alone.
Head	Headaches and migraine.
Face	Nasal catarrh, clear or white discharge. Nasal ulceration with bleeding. Corneal ulceration. Flushing and heat during headaches.
Abdomen	Marked flatulence with abdominal distension. Borborygmi Indigestion. Tender liver. Jaundice.
Appetite	Desires eggs, sweets, salt and hot food. < eggs, fats.
Cardiovascular	Palpitations < night. Discomfort around heart.
Urogenital	Renal calculi. Pyelitis and nephritis accompanied by colic. Headaches linked to genital function, especially at menopause. Premenstral tension.
Respiratory	Nasal catarrh.
Musculoskeletal	Rheumatism and arthritis. Pain under shoulder blades especially on right. Loss of power in limbs.
Sleep	Poor. Palpitations may wake.
Skin	Pruritis. Psoriasis.
Modalities & Generals	< 4–8 pm. < heat, night, eating. > movement.

CASE 5.1   A non-specific pruritis

A bowel nosode, selected on broad principles, in fact proves to be the required remedy.

A four-year-old entire male Saluki was presented with generalised pruritis. He had been bred by the present owners and was one of four in the household. Two of these were related, one being his mother and another being his brother. The other dog, a male, had been bought as a puppy some two years previously and was not closely related. All four got on well together and there was no obvious pecking order. His brother was very boisterous, and the owners felt that at times his sheer enthusiasm was resented by the others, especially by the patient. At such times the patient would give a half-hearted bite and move away from his brother, but there never appeared to be any serious resentment or attempt to fight. None of the dogs had suffered from any skin problems in the past and there was no sign of any problems in the other three at the time of the first consultation.

The dog was not nervous of noise. He spent most of the time with the other dogs in an outdoor kennel and run, and only came into the house in the evenings. At such times he was happy to be inside but took care to avoid any source of heat. On the other hand he would not actively seek the coolest spot that he could find, but was quite happy to lie in the middle of the room. When outside he appeared not to be upset by the sun but would lie in its direct beam; really hot weather did not appear to distress him. He appeared to enjoy physical fussing if it was offered to him although he never sought it and was not jealous when it was given to any of the others. His appetite was described as 'average' but what food he had was always eaten very quickly, to the extent that he would occasionally vomit soon after-wards. When this happened he would immediately eat the vomited food again with no ill effects. The diet, in common with the other dogs, consisted of commercially prepared food. The quantity drunk was difficult to quantify as there was a communal supply in the outside run. However, he was the only one of the four who ever drank in the house, and when he did he would take a long drink. He was never offered milk. His bowels were usually normal.

He was happy to go outside, either on his own or with the others. He was not particular about keeping himself clean and would run through puddles, mud and wet grass without a second thought. He disliked rain, was impervious to wind, and had no objection to walking in snow. He had been shown and had performed 'adequately'; he had no dislike of being bathed and groomed for show purposes and there had been no adverse effects on the skin from the process. When being taken to a show he travelled well, and that was the only occasion when he went in a car, except for visits to a vet.

He had suffered no previous major health problems, the only events being the occasional minor cut and strain. All had resolved either without treatment or with short courses of conventional treat-ment. He had been vaccinated as a puppy at ten and twelve weeks of age, receiving a booster at eighteen months and another at thirty months without any observed reaction to any of them. He was wormed routinely with the other dogs using a prescription preparation.

The present trouble had started some nine weeks prior to the consultation, when redness and irritation had appeared for no apparent reason on both front legs below the knees (wrists) and between the toes. This had been diagnosed as a contact allergy, although to what was never established. Treatment was with the steroid prednisolone by mouth, which quickly removed the irritation but had no effect on the redness. A few days after the end of the course of prednisolone the irritation returned and the affected area began to spread up and round the legs. The owner administered a self-prescribed herbal shampoo that was ineffective and the condition continued to spread rapidly over the whole body and the hind legs. There was generalised irritation with deep red patches on all four feet, around the base of the tail and in the right axilla and groin.

Another visit to the vet for conventional treatment resulted in the administration of systemic as well as oral steroids, plus a course of antibiotic (Synulox) and a medicated shampoo (Malaseb). This again gave temporary relief from the pruritis but did not affect the appearance or distribution of the lesions. Skin scrapes were negative for all ectoparasites and mites. The pruritis returned after the end of the treatment and at this point homeopathic help was sought.

On examination the skin was dry and there were no discharges. The only breaks in the skin were self-inflicted and some had been bleeding. Nibbling and scratching were continuous, and even exercise did not take the dog's mind off the irritation. He would stop in mid-run to attack himself. The redness varied from a bright red to a deep almost purple hue in the longest standing areas. There was no heat in the skin at any point and no excessive or abnormal smell. In line with the previous examinations there was no sign of any ectoparasites. Although the picture was not one normally associated with ringworm infection, a culture test was carried out that proved negative. Neither the ears nor the anal glands were affected. The dog's appetite had not been affected in any way. His thirst had not changed even when he was receiving steroids.

Treatment was commenced with Morgan Bach in the 30c potency, to be given night and morning for four days. Re-examination three weeks later showed that the irritation on the body had virtually ceased and had also considerably reduced on the legs. There had been no change in the discolouration of the skin. The owners felt that the improvement had been steady for about eight or nine days after starting the remedy, but it had then ceased and had subsequently regressed slightly. There had been no change in the dog's general demeanour. The Morgan Bach was repeated, but this time in the 200c potency, night and morning for two days. After a further three weeks the body was completely clear and the discolourations in the axilla and groin were fading. Those on the legs, however, were the same and there was still a moderate degree of irritation associated with them. The owner felt that the improvement had once more plateaued and hence a further prescription of Morgan Bach 200c morning, night and morning for three doses was administered. Progress was then resumed and after another ten days the axilla and groin were completely clear and although the discolouration on the legs was still there it was generally fading and there was no irritation. No further prescription was made and one month later everything had settled apart from some deep areas of discolouration between the front toes. Three doses of Morgan Bach 200c as above were repeated, following which every-thing settled down and there have been no further troubles.

Discussion

This was a case where, in a sense, the remedy was right for the wrong reason. The management of the dog, which is not uncommon in the veterinary world, introduced constraints on the amount of detailed infor-mation that could be obtained from the owners. The initial consultation had revealed some pointers towards a number of remedies, but with no strong indication for any one. Whilst there was an obvious link to the skin, there was no previous history to suggest any underlying condition as a possible aetiology. The redness of the skin, the intense irritation and the disregard for weather conditions and dirt suggested Sulphur, although there was no smell, marked heat connection or adverse reaction to bathing. Simi-larly, the fact of continuing pruritis during exercise suggested possibly Graphites or Arsenicum Album, but nothing else in the case fitted either remedy. The only link to Psorinum was the liking for heat, but even this was ambivalent. It will never be known what the effect of giving Sulphur would have been, and it is likely that there would have been some positive effect. However, Morgan Bach was decided upon primarily on the basis of the skin connection of the symptoms. The subsequent progress of the case showed this to be the correct remedy from the simillimum point of view, with the steady progress of the case and no other remedy being required. If Sulphur had in fact been the correct remedy, the effect of the bowel nosode would have been to produce a changed symptom picture with stronger indications for Sulphur, whose administration as the second prescription would have taken the case forward. In view of the nature of the remedy as the correct choice rather than as a clearing remedy, the dosage regime became that of the simillimum rather than following the protocols for the other used of the bowel remedies.

CASE 5.2   An unexpected twist

A well indicated remedy takes the case forward to a considerable degree, but the presenting symptom yields finally to the appropriate bowel nosode.

A fifty-six year-old lady was suffering from persistent migraines. She had experienced the occasional attack since she was a teenager, with a gradual worsening through her adult life. Over the past six years they had increased markedly in both frequency and intensity follow-ing a car accident whilst on holiday in Europe, in which she sustained a whiplash injury. She had taken Arnica at the time of the accident and had received several courses of chiropractic treatment since. There had been at best a temporary beneficial effect and the situation now was that the attacks were occurring almost weekly, with sudden onset, and lasting for up to thirty-six hours. She was completely incapacitated by them and even when they had passed she felt completely 'washed out'. The headaches started on the right side and spread over the whole head: she described the feeling 'as if there is a brick inside my head', and at the worst times she was unable to lift her head from the pillow. There was a sensation of a tight band around the forehead accompanied by feelings of nausea. During a migraine there was a sensation of too much light entering the right eye, even when shut. Full investigations, including scans, had revealed no abnormalities.

The lady was married with an unmarried adult son and a married daughter, all in their thirties. Together with her husband all five worked in a successful family business, which involved a heavy workload with periods of very hectic activity.. Her main tasks involved the running of the office and general backup services for the staff. The husband, who was the same age as she was, wanted to ease out and leave the day-to- day running of the business to their children, a move that she supported, and wished to join him in a more leisured lifestyle. Both liked to take regular holidays. The children, however, whilst working hard and loyally, were unwilling to take on that ultimate responsibility. This she found both annoying and worrying as far as the long-term future was concerned. Neither she nor her husband wished to retire completely, and she, whilst enjoying what time she took away from the business, admitted to feeling guilty if she did not go in to work regularly. This, however, only applied if she took the odd day off and never if she went away on holiday. Her eldest son had suffered from respiratory problems for the previous ten years and there had been several major but unfounded scares during that time. Her husband's father died of cancer, and she herself was fearful of the condition. As a consequence she constantly worried about the health of all the family. All, of necessity, lived locally to her and although she loved them all, including her son-in-law, she nevertheless enjoyed time away from them.

Her family medical history was unremarkable. Apart from the worsening migraines, since the accident she had experienced irregular tingling sensations in both arms, but especially the left. She had a longstanding tendency to colds and occasional sinus problems, but an ENT specialist had recommended no treatment. She had experienced some cardiac arrhythmia about fifteen years previously, but investigations had revealed nothing. No treatment had been given and the symptoms resolved with no further problems.

The consultation revealed that she enjoyed both company and being on her own. She liked open spaces and adored living on the side of a hill with long vistas across a valley. She was keen on her garden but found that she quickly became hot when working in it (she did not do any heavy digging). She tended to do everything quickly, always wanting to get on to the next job and needing to be active all the time. She had no significant fears. She loved colour, bright sunlight and dancing provided that the music was quick. Although not seeking great heat she liked to be warm, and her hands and feet would quickly become cold, even in summer. When alone she would always have music on the radio, and would sing and dance along to any lively tune. She did not sleep well and when she dreamt it was usually of either water or dead relatives.

She preferred cold food, especially salads, honey and tomatoes, and was not keen on sweets. She loved vinegar to the extent of being willing to drink it. She was not enthusiastic about salt, never using it in cooking, but being willing to eat food prepared with it in a social situation. There were no other food desires and her only real hate was for whisky, even disliking its smell.

The remedy selected was Sepia on the basis of her mental symptoms and reactions to her situation, and the general and local symptoms surrounding activity, food and circulation. It was given as a 30c night and morning for three days. Five days after the consultation the lady went on a two week holiday to Spain with her husband and there was a second homeopathic consultation two weeks after her return. Two days after the outward flight there had been another attack as bad as before, but after that there had been nothing until just before coming home. This latter, however, was milder and although it lasted nearly twenty-four hours she was able, as she described it, to 'live through it'.

Two days after her return she had attended for a routine health check under her health insurance scheme. At that check a heart irregularity was found of which she had been completely unaware. Following tests the consultant recommended treatment with betablockers, which she declined.

She admitted to being worried by the heart findings and had suffered from a nagging headache for about two days after the health check. However, there had been no more full migraine attacks and she described herself as feeling 'normal' in spite of having moderate headaches fairly frequently. It was decided to wait until after her next consultation with the heart consultant before considering any further homeopathic treatment. A week later she had what was classified as a 'moderate' migraine attack.

The follow-up heart consultation showed that her heart now appeared clinically normal and a further prescription of Sepia was given, this time at 200c, three doses over twenty-four hours. Another ECG after three months was again normal. At this time she was having headaches every three to four weeks but no migraines. The frequency continued to decline without further treatment over the next four to five months until all regular headaches ceased, with the only occurrences being linked to periods of high business stress over deadlines to be met. These were of short duration when they did occur and never seemed likely to develop into a migraine. This remained the picture for some eleven months, at the end of which time a very bad migraine struck again – 'one of the worst I have ever had', with tension down the back of the neck, nausea, intense photophobia and thumping in the head. Morgan Bach 1M was given and the attack began to ease about half an hour after the first dose. A further dose was given after another two hours and one final one twelve hours later. This completely resolved the situation and all has remained well for the past two years. A further routine health check for insurance purposes revealed no heart worries.

Discussion

The choice of remedy in this case appeared clear-cut, and in view of that a higher potency could possibly have been used initially. This may have given a better result and avoided the need to move up the potencies as was necessary. The instruction to always use a clearly indicated remedy in preference to a bowel nosode (Paterson J.) was followed and the response to treatment confirmed the choice. The re-appearance of the old symptom of cardiac irregularity was an example of Hering's Law and its subsequent disappearance without treatment fits the pattern. The final use of Morgan Bach, and the higher potency employed, was indicated on the keynote of the great cerebral congestion at that time and the acute nature of the attack, but since it resolved the whole case there was obviously a deeper aspect that was also addressed. Morgan Bach was used as there was no clear indication in the case pointing to either of the other two Morgan nosodes. It should also be noted that whilst Sepia is among the associated remedies of both Morgan Pure and Morgan Gaertner, it is not a leading remedy of either group (see Chapter 2), although in the modern expanded list it is in the second degree in relation to Morgan Pure (see Appendix). Sepia is also an associated remedy of Proteus, which might have seemed the more obvious choice of nosode with the sudden onset and the nervous involvement, but the congestive theme symptom dictated quite clearly another direction. Equally, although there were undoubtedly periods of stress in this lady's situation, there was not the continuous stress, more usually associated with Proteus.

CASE 5.3   Remedy choice within a group

The use of a bowel nosode indicated by the remedies employed previously unlocks the full effect of an indicated remedy.

An eight-year-old male African grey parrot, suffering from persistent swelling and redness of both jowels extending to the commissures of the mouth, was referred from a specialist exotic animal practice. The lesions were essentially non-irritant and there was no marked difference in intensity between the two sides of the face. The problem had appeared some eighteen months previously with no obvious cause. The diagnosis was 'chronic hyperplasic lymphocytic/plastacytic perivascular dermatitis'. All blood parameters were within normal limits and dermatophyte culture had been negative. The findings of a biopsy taken from the left side some three months previously had been interpreted by the laboratory as being 'typical of hypersensitive responses in birds', although further comments in the report cast doubts on whether allergic skin disease does in fact exist in birds. Treatment had been with antibiotics and antihistamines. Various diet combinations and changes of perch material had been tried but these had produced no beneficial effect.

At the consultation the bird was in good general health. On a scale from 0 (perfect) to 10 (very bad), the owner estimated the severity of the condition at 4: the worst it had ever been was 6. The bird was very attached to his female owner, responding positively on her approach and interacting with her. The lady's partner, however, received no such affection although there was never any sign of any aggression. Strangers were viewed with caution, and if such a person were near the cage the bird would come to its front only if the lady were present as well. Generally he would come out of his cage only if the lady was present, and occasionally he would refuse to come out even for her. He was never offered the chance to come out in the presence of strangers but the lady did not think he would ever do that. His appetite was good and catholic. Motions were normal and had not been upset by any of the diet changes that had been tried. He never emptied his water container completely and had a definite liking for milk.

Although the constitutional type is not as easy to determine in birds as in mammals, the combination of timidity and affection when compared to the species norm suggested Pulsatilla. In view of the chronic nature of the problem it was decided to use the chronic of

Pulsatilla, which also fitted the picture to some extent plus the inflammatory element that was present. The owner was able to administer medication directly to the bird in a drop of milk, and treatment was begun with Silica LM1 for two weeks. The treatment resulted in a steady although limited improvement with the severity varying between 2 and 3 on the owner's scale after three weeks. There was then a regression with intermittent flaring of the condition with considerable redness and some irritation of the affected areas.

The condition now resembled a more typical mammalian allergic reaction. In spite of the doubts expressed in the laboratory report as to whether true allergic reactions in fact do occur in birds, the appearance of the lesions were so typical that a possible allergic basis for the condition could not be ignored. Tuberculinum Bovinum 200c was accordingly given night and morning for two days. This produced an improvement to the extent that the acute episodes ceased, although the swelling and some redness remained. The liking for milk was now considered to a greater extent than previously, together with the rest of the picture, and consequently Rhus Tox. 200c was given night and morning for four days. Following this the owner estimated a consistent severity of 2 on her scale, which was maintained but not improved on. Morgan Pure 200c night and morning for four days was then prescribed. For the first time there was complete resolution of the problem for one week, followed by a slight regression. The severity now continued to vary slightly but the owner's estimate was of a maximum degree of 1. In addition she remarked that 'I can't put my finger on it but somehow he seems more alert'.

After a month the situation was unchanged and Morgan Pure was given again, three doses over twenty-four hours at a potency of 1M, without obvious effect. It was decided to revert to the original remedy and Silica 200c night and morning for two days was administered. The skin cleared and remained so for eleven months, at which time the problem appeared to be returning. Three doses of Silica 200c over twenty-four hours were given and all settled once more. Contact was lost some eighteen months later when the owner left the country, but up to that time there had been no further problems.

Discussion

The patient in this case was of a species not usually associated with the bowel nosodes, and one in which the digestive physiology is different from the mammalian. Nevertheless, it is clear that the Morgan Pure fitted into the treatment regime following the same underlying principles as govern the use of the bowel nosodes in other species. This emphasises the fact that the concept underlying the bowel nosodes represents a universal and fundamental natural healing function at the deepest level.

In Chapter 3 (pages 36–38) the use of a bowel nosode as a means of clarifying a symptom picture has been described. This case was in some ways the reverse of that. With the sequence of remedies used, all chosen on the presenting clinical picture, the reactions produced identifying the necessary bowel nosode. All the remedies produced some beneficial effect although none gave the final breakthrough. However, all three are represented in the associated remedies of Morgan Pure (as is Pulsatilla, which had a role in the thinking process for the initial remedy selection). In addition, Morgan Pure has an affinity with the skin. However, it is interesting that even though the bowel nosode gave the final leap towards cure, it was not of itself the complete answer. The bowel nosode had the effect of enhancing the action of the Silica, the initially chosen remedy, thereby allowing it to complete its work.

The choice of potency was influenced by the higher metabolic rate of birds compared to mammals, hence the use of 200c as standard. The LM potency was used because of the history of medication and the desire to commence treatment with a longer course of treatment than would be used generally with a centesimal potency.

CASE 5.4   The depth of dis-ease

A chance injury produces a stubborn symptom that is linked to the underlying imbalance in the patient, and which is resolved finally by the use of a bowel nosode addressing that imbalance.

A fifty-two-year-old married lady had the misfortune to trip off the edge of a pavement and land awkwardly, sustaining a partial fracture of the fifth metatarsal of the left foot, together with soft tissue damage around the ankle. Arnica 1M was administered immediately and, following x-ray examination, external fixation by means of a surgical boot was established. Bone density was identified as normal. Symphytum 30c was taken once daily for two weeks and twice weekly after that. After one month further x-rays showed satisfactory healing; the boot was discarded and the Symphytum ceased. Unfortunately, at this stage circumstances dictated that the lady was obliged to walk on the foot more than was desirable. This was possible but painful, and considerable soft tissue swelling of the whole foot resulted from this use. The swelling went down with rest but there was always some discomfort present and great sensitivity to the slightest pressure. Apis Mel. and Ruta Grav., both at 30c, did not relieve the situation to any significant degree but Phytolacca and Calc Fluor. at the same potency helped considerably over the next month. At this stage the lady was able to rest the leg more, but the tendency to a degree of swelling persisted. The situation improved slowly over the next six weeks, aided by physiotherapy, but had not resolved at the end of that time. There was still a degree of constant discomfort in the foot and it continued to be larger than its companion to the extent that she was considerably restricted as to what shoes she could wear.

As far as was known her childhood history was unremarkable. At the age of thirty-two she had suffered an inflammatory condition of the gall bladder, resulting in removal of that organ. Eight years later there was an acute illness diagnosed as hepatitis, although no causal organism was isolated. Since then there had been a tendency to eczema, especially behind the ears, that responded to Graphites 30c. The gall bladder problem had left a legacy of intolerance to fats, with a tendency to flatulence and burning in the oesophagus if too much was eaten. The flatulence had at times been present, independent of fats, and appeared to be triggered by any abnormally large intake of food. Arsenicum Album had helped the problem to some extent whereas Lycopodium proved of no benefit. She enjoyed all travel and new experiences, and had a very definite sense of right and wrong. She had difficulty in delegating in her job, and demanded an orderly working environment. She enjoyed heat but disliked a stuffy atmosphere. Her appetite was of average size but she quickly felt full. There was a desire for spices and savoury tastes, fruit and vegetables. The only marked dislike was for milk and milk products. Thirst was unremarkable, and although she insisted on her food always being very hot she disliked hot liquids. At the time of the injury all her digestive symptoms were in abeyance.

Although the sensitivity of the foot to pressure continued at all times, the particular pain and the presence of the swelling had settled into a definite pattern. Irrespective of the degree of use during the day, the swelling always worsened in the early evening and the pain intensified on the sole of the foot. There was no undue heat associated with the symptoms. Applying ice to the affected area eased the situation but elevating the foot did not. Invariably the swelling had disappeared by next morning.

Morgan Gaertner 30c was prescribed, night and morning for three doses. Both the pain and the swelling resolved within one week, but the pain began to return after a further ten days. A single dose of Morgan Gaertner at 200c was administered, the pain regressed, and did not return. The foot returned to its normal size and the choice of shoes became unrestricted once more. After this there was a return of the flatulence and oesophageal burning. No treatment was given and the symptoms disappeared over two weeks. The foot remained normal except for some aching after extensive use. General health has remained good, with no recurrence of the eczema.

Discussion

This case emphasises the importance of taking the full medical history into account. The initial treatment of the injury had been concentrated very much at the local level, and had certainly helped to a considerable degree. The fracture may well have healed satisfactorily without Symphytum, but the success of the Phytolacca and Calc Fluor. would indicate that there had been some significant damage to the ligaments and/or tendons as well as the bone damage. The persistent swelling did not appear to be linked to any acute inflammatory process as there was never any heat in the area. Equally, at the end there did not seem to be any relationship between the degree of swelling and the amount of use of the foot. There was obviously some passive congestion remaining in the area, possibly as a result of local damage to the circulation, although there was never any temperature variation in the feet.

What was significant, however, was the time aggravation of the symptoms. The early evening aggravation was very marked and pointed towards Lycopodium, Chelidonium or Morgan Gaertner as possible remedies. The history of inflammatory involvement of both gall bladder and liver, together with the passive congestion and the time modality indicated the nosode.

It would appear that the use of the bowel nosode addressed the deeper 'dis-ease' that was present in this patient. Graphites is an associated remedy of Morgan Gaertner, although it is interesting to note that Lycopodium had produced no clinical benefit when given.

6

DYSENTERY CO.

Traditionally associated remedies
Anacardium Or, Argent Nit, **Arsenicum Alb**, Cadmium Met, Kalmia Lat,
Veratrum Alb, Veratrum Vir.

General considerations

The indications for this nosode are not found as commonly as with the
Morgan group, but it is nevertheless of major clinical value. In his general
survey John Paterson found the NLFB associated with Dysentery Co. in
1.77% of his samples and Elizabeth Paterson found them in 4.24% of her
cases. Although none of the NLFB were found in the animal survey, there
is no doubt that the nosode is of equally significant use in animals. The
generally quoted theme of 'anticipatory anxiety' should be thought of more
as a broader 'nervous tension' with an emphasis on its anticipatory aspects
(Boyd 1989). The nosode has the themes of stress, anxiety and insecurity
running through it, resulting in an inability to relax. The major miasmatic
aspects of the nosodes are sycotic and syphilitic.

Dysentery Co. was the first of the bowel nosodes to be clearly identified
(Dishington 1929) regarding both the NLFB of the group and the materia
medica of the nosode. It must be stressed that the bowel nosode is not
connected with the acute clinical conditions classed as dysentery but
should be considered where there is a history of 'never well since' acute
dysenteric attacks (Paterson). It is very much associated with anticipatory
anxiety, the sort of worry that 'hits in the solar plexus'. John Paterson
defined the theme as 'nervous tension' (1953), and either fear or excitement
will bring on or aggravate symptoms. The individual requiring the nosode
is indeed usually a nervous type who faces any duty or task with trepida-
tion. The worry arises on two fronts, either an anticipation of what might
go wrong and hence a fear of failure, or a concern that they will fall short
of the high standards they have set themselves (Paterson 1953). There is

no fear of complete failure in either of these reactions. Arsenicum Album, the leading remedy of the group, shows this very clearly in the 'perfectionist' aspect of its picture, summed up in the phrase 'anything worth doing is worth overdoing'. (The reader is referred to Catherine Coulter's *Portraits of Homoeopathic remedies* vol. 1 for a complete discussion of this aspect of Arsenicum). The source of the nervous tension found in the type is thus essentially intrinsic. The perfectionist desire leads to over-worry and overwork, with consequent functional upsets to the circulatory and endocrine systems. This shows as thyroid problems, physical exhaustion and temperature control failures. The (thoroughbred) horse is often described as the typical Arsenicum type (Clarke 1982). Argentum Nitricum is also often quoted as being a very typical remedy of the group, as is Kalmia (Paterson 1948), and it is perhaps surprising that these two are not routinely classified more highly than the first degree in the associated remedies. In fact, in his 1948 address to the British Homoeopathic Congress, John Paterson listed Kalmia as being on an equal level to Arsenicum Album among the associated remedies and in his 1953 paper he reiterates that the three main remedies associated with Dysentery Co. are Arsenicum Album, Argentum Nitricum and Kalmia. Also in the same 1948 address he raises the possibility of a link between Lycopodium and the nosode, and Lycopodium has been shown to follow Dysentery Co. well. The main areas of action for Dysentery Co are the nervous system, the duodenum and the heart. Cardiac conditions of nervous origin call for its use (Agrawal 1995). It is indicated in cases of duodenal ulcers that arise following a period of anxiety accompanied by feelings of tension in the stomach and heart regions, and the ulcers are often seen in young individuals who are of an essentially nervous temperament. Racehorses, who are by definition young, live lives of stress and high expectations, and gastric ulcers are a commonly found condition, with up to 100% of some stables being affected (Conwell 2009). It is no surprise that Dysentery Co., together with Proteus (Chapter 6), are both major remedies for the upper alimentary ulcers that such horses develop (Armstrong 2007). It also proved to be of particular use in children (Paterson 1937); it has proved successful against sleeplessness in children when caused by anxiety about examinations or other school linked events such as sporting fixtures, where the patient's worry centres around their ability to perform well. Similarly, the nosode in its own right can be used in animals that do not perform well in the show ring (the two remedies used most commonly, Argentum Nit. and Gelsemium are both present in the associated remedy group for Dysentery Co.). Cyclical vomiting in highly strung individuals has been responsive (Foubister 1988). Pyloric stenosis due to spasm from nervous tension will usually respond (Paterson

1953). It should be considered in cases of chorea and nervous tics generally and migraine of nervous origin may respond (Agrawal 1995).

Dysentery Co. has connections with adult onset allergies such as hay fever and rhinitis, and there is a tendency towards a general hypersensitivity. Low-grade inflammatory conditions of the respiratory tract are seen.

Materia medica

There is a possible aetiology of infection, especially when linked to the excessive use of antibiotics. All symptoms tend to be worse when in a warm room.

The mental picture is one of nervousness, anxiety and excitability, especially in situations involving new events or people. This may show as fear and avoidance of company, whilst at the other extreme there can be fear of being alone. There can be great insecurity and lack of self-confidence. Obsessive Compulsive Disorder can be seen. A general aggravation from crowds is a feature. The type is generally fearful and will quickly get minor matters out of proportion – always 'making a crisis out of a drama'. The anxiety about performance leads to the individual being extremely sensitive to criticism, and this can result in outbursts of violent anger. The general mental state is expressed as restlessness and an inability to remain still, resulting in impatience and with everything being done quickly, and an inability to relax. The type is aggravated by consolation. There is a general sensitivity to all external stimuli. In dogs this is seen as the animal that is hypersensitive to noise, fearful of it unless its source can be located and barking excessively at the slightest provocation (for example, every time the telephone rings). Frontal headaches can be severe and tend to occur on a regular time pattern, usually within a framework of seven to fourteen days. Blepharitis, styes and conjunctivitis with sticky discharges are accompanied by functional upsets to vision, either with or without headache. The face is a major area for muscular tics and twitches. There are purulent discharges from the ears, with sudden swelling and inflammation.

The general tension affects the digestive system, causing chronic indigestion with flatulence and heartburn and the symptomatology is linked particularly to the upper gastrointestinal tract around the pylorus and duodenum. The nosode shares the Arsenicum Album modality of being worse around midnight to 1.00 a.m. In Dysentery Co. this takes the form of waking with acute pain in the stomach relieved by vomiting mucus, and waking later in the night (3 to 4 a.m.) with abdominal pain also occurs. Conditions are generally worse for eating, giving feelings of fullness and bloating in both stomach and abdomen, and there may be severe pain especially on the right side. However, eating can give relief to a gnawing emptiness in the stomach. There is a desire for sweets, milk, fats, cheese and salt, with aggravation from fats and sweets. Also seen is a desire for cold drinks, but the stomach is aggravated by them. Diarrhoea and constipation are both seen. Diarrhoea occurs in the morning with forcible passage of mucoid stool and frequent motions throughout the day. The constipation shows either unproductive straining or the passage of small hard stools, again with mucus. Sharp cutting pains are felt when passing a motion.

The state of tension appears in the cardiovascular system as functional disturbances of the heart action with palpitations and discomfort in the chest, especially before any event and after food. Tachycardia and irregular beats are seen, with pains extending around the left shoulder and down the left arm. Exertion aggravates the cardiac symptoms, giving a poor exercise tolerance. There is involvement of the veins, with dilation and stasis leading to varicose veins, easy bleeding, bruising and a tendency for dilation of the veins, giving overheating of the head. The poor circulation gives swellings, coldness and numbness of both hands and feet. The stasis associated with the circulation means that there is a general desire for heat linked to a dislike of stuffy atmosphere, causing nausea and faintness. The skin is often pale due to a combination of feeble circulation and a degree of anaemia. The type perspires easily on exertion but also just with excitement, whilst skin symptoms may be produced as a result of either excitement or fear. The skin is dry and scaly and the head may be most markedly affected.

The respiratory system shows a shortness of breath and poor exercise tolerance. Paroxysmal cough, bronchial catarrh and lung consolidation are found. There are feelings of suffocation, especially at night with great desire to take a deep breath. The nosode's general modality of being worse between 3–6 a.m. shows particularly in the respiratory system.

In the female there is dysmenorrhoea. Pelvic pain and irritation of both vagina and vulva are seen. Pain is felt in the bladder before passing water, with burning in the urethra afterwards. Travelling stimulates the need to pass water.

The musculoskeletal system exhibits muscular twitches and feelings of tightness in muscles. Nails are of poor quality with easily infected, painful nail beds. Neuralgic pains extend down legs and arms. Rheumatism of the jaw, neck and shoulders with stiffness, and arthritis of the knees and feet are seen. Conditions are accompanied by great pain, especially of the spine.

The skin discharges are sticky (cf. Graphites) and tend to dry to crusts. There is cracking of the skin which heals – this then breaks down again continuously. The skin is predominantly dry and flaky and scales occur in the flexures of joints. Some warts are to be found.

Sleep is often poor with many unpleasant dreams. There is difficulty in getting to sleep due to an overactive mind, accompanied by cardiac palpitations.

DYSENTERY CO.	
Mind	Nervous. Anxious and insecure. Excitable. Lack of confidence in new situations. Resents criticism. Restless. Phobias.
Head	Frontal headaches following a regular pattern.
Face	Muscle twitches. Inflammatory conditions of the eyes. Upsets to vision. Purulent discharges from ears.
Abdomen	Chronic indigestion. Flatulence. Duodenal ulcers. Pyloric stenosis. Pain in both stomach and intestines especially on right side. Feeling of fullness in abdomen. <eating. Mucus on stools. Forceful diarrhoea in morning. Constipation with unproductive straining.
Appetite	Desires sweets, milk, fats, cheese and salt. Desires cold drinks but stomach <. <fats and sweets.
Cardiovascular	Anticipatory palpitations with discomfort in chest. Tachycardia. Pain down left arm. Poor exercise tolerance. Poor circulation.
Urogenital	Urination while travelling. Pain in bladder before urination. Pelvic pain. Dysmenorrhoea. Irritation of vulva and vagina.
Respiratory	Shortness of breath. Paroxysmal cough. Bronchial catarrh. Asthma and Hay fever.
Musculoskeletal	Muscular twitches. Tightness in muscles. Rheumatism of shoulders and neck. Conditions show great pain. Neuralgias.
Sleep	Sleepless through mental activity. Palpitations on falling asleep. Unpleasant dreams.
Skin	Warts. Sticky discharges. Skin breaks down easily.
Modalities & Generalities	A chilly remedy. Sensitive to stimuli. < 3–6 a.m., crowds, consolation, eating. > Warmth, open air.

CASE 6.1   Getting to the root of fear

Various remedies are prescribed over time to address different manifestations of an underlying fear. It is only when the bowel nosode associated with the most successful of these is given that the final cure is obtained.

A crossbred female terrier, estimated at ten years of age, had arrived with her present owners, a married couple, when she was approximately two years old, having been re-homed from a stray kennel at that time. Nothing was known of her history prior to entering the kennels, but whilst there she had been both neutered and vaccinated. The owners had an adult daughter who lived nearby with a handicapped son, and the couple were closely involved in his care. The presenting problem was one of generalised pruritis of varying intensity, but with no periods of complete freedom from irritation. This irritation had been present at the time of the adoption, with no skin lesions or other indication of skin disease. It had been described as 'a nervous itch that will stop as soon as she is in a stable home'. There had been no other signs of any clinical conditions when she had been re-homed, and subsequently there had been no health problems other than those associated with the pruritis. The dog had indeed settled into her new home but at no time had the pruritis ceased completely. It was always there to some extent, with an acute flare-up being precipitated by any shock or upset in routine. Such events were usually accompanied by explosive and urgent diarrhoea. No blood or mucus was seen in the stool. At such times she would eat grass but there was no excessive flatulence. The attacks lasted for about two days and were not accompanied by any signs of systemic illness. The dog had received booster vaccinations for the initial three years in her current home, with no observed reactions, but these had then been stopped. Over the years she had been wormed 'two or three times' with prescribed agents. There were several semi-feral cats in the neighbourhood in addition to a cat in the household, and routine flea treatment was accordingly being given. The only other medications had been steroids and antihistamines for the skin problem. The antihistamines had produced no effect and the steroids only temporary alleviation. There had been no changes to appetite or thirst as a result of the steroids.

On examination the skin appeared cool and dry with some flaky scabs. There were no open sores, and never had been. The ears were clear and had never been involved in the problem. The weight was 9.8kg and, in view of the fine-boned build of the dog, was considered normal. Thirst and appetite were unremarkable. She was fed on chicken and fish, as it had been found that red meat aggravated the skin. Similarly, if she stole the cat's tinned food this too adversely affected the skin. Vegetables would not be eaten but there was a liking for apples, pears and grapes.

The temperament was described as lively. There was a great attachment to the wife, who would be followed round the house at all times. A general liking to be near people was evident, linked to a dislike of being closely cuddled or restrained. She was friendly to strangers after exhibiting an initial wariness to any new contact, either human or animal. The household's cat was largely ignored. In the home environment the dog was calm but became easily restless and agitated in strange surroundings. She was sensitive to all sound; during the day she would not be upset by it but at night she became disturbed and began to bark. In the consulting room she would not settle but was constantly trying to find a way out. There was no aggression on being examined but she was trying to get away all the time whilst shaking and refusing to make eye contact. There was a definite fear of thunder and fireworks. Even a mild storm would produce looseness of the bowels, and a severe one would trigger an aggravation of the pruritis. She was not keen to go out in wind or rain even for a walk, which in other conditions she enjoyed greatly. She would walk in snow but showed no inclination to play in it. She was obsessive about being clean and any dirt was licked off immediately. She liked heat generally, and would seek a source such as a fire or radiator. In summer she would lie out in the sun and in winter would lie in shafts of sunlight coming through windows.

Arsenicum Album 30c, night and morning for five days, was prescribed on the basis of the general liveliness, the desire for security with fear and restlessness, especially at night, the love of heat, the dryness of the skin and the desire to be clean. This resulted in a complete resolution of the skin symptoms for one year. During that time there had been occasional bouts of looseness but even these had not been as severe as previously. After that time the pruritis returned to its original pattern. The return of the symptoms had occurred shortly after the death of the owner's grandson. The dog had apparently been very attached to him and had been distraught at his death, together with the consequent upset in the whole family. The Ars Alb. was repeated as above. The condition settled once more but only for some six weeks. At this time there was intense irritation that eased with scratching; the skin felt hot but was not red and many dry flaky scabs appeared on the back. The area around the hind quarters were worst affected, and there was now excessive hair loss but no alopecia. The anal glands were impacted but not infected; these were expressed manually and a course of Silica 30c night and morning for four days was given. This resolved the acute situation and the skin reverted to exhibiting only a slight irritation. All remained well for a further three months until the start of the build-up to the English celebrations of Guy Fawkes on November 5th. The resultant increasing outbursts of fireworks over the period produced a slight increase in the pruritis, but mainly a marked increase in the diarrhoea. Abdominal investigations revealed no abnormality. The other change was a significant increase in the sensitivity to noise. Phosphorus 30c night and morning was prescribed for five days. However, after three doses the skin became markedly worse; accordingly the remedy was stopped and the skin improved. At the same time the sensitivity to noise eased but as the 'firework season' itself was now easing this was difficult to interpret.

Over the next two years there were a total of four flare-ups of the skin, all of which responded to Ars Alb. However, it was becoming necessary to increase the potency to 200c in order to obtain the benefit. Some five months after the last of these a series of severe storms with much thunder triggered a really acute state with much distress for the dog, together with pruritis and diarrhoea. Aconite 10M was prescribed for 'emergency' use, followed by Ars Alb. again at 30c night and morning for three days. The diarrhoea eased but the skin was not relieved, the picture changing to one of redness with some heat and a definite aggravation from heat. Sulphur 30c night and morning for three days removed all symptoms except the pruritis, which persisted.

At this stage Dysentery Co was prescribed, 30c night and morning for four days. Three weeks later the skin had settled completely and the dog was reported as being 'very happy in herself'. The wife had been away for two days during the time and there had been no suspicion of any relapse. All remained clear until four months later until the 'firework season' came round again. This caused some obvious mental distress, slight pruritis, but no diarrhoea. Dysentery Co. was administered night and morning for three days at 200c and all was resolved. There have been no further problems for the past five years.

Discussion

The management of this case was influenced by having, at various stages, the input of three veterinary surgeons, of whom one was the author. However, its pattern also demonstrates how progress can be diverted by concentrating on too specific aspects of the picture and prescribing accordingly. Arsenicum Album was clearly the constitutional remedy for this dog and its initial prescription produced a good response. The trigger for the first relapse, the death of the owners' grandson, could have led to the use of remedies such as Ignatia or Nat Mur. with their association with grief and bereavement. However, it was felt that the dog's reaction was linked more to the general upset in her environment than to specific grieving. This, together with the good response to the initial prescription, indicated a repetition of the remedy, and initially this appeared justified. The subsequent change to Silica rather that an increase in the potency of the Arsenicum was dictated by the changed presenting picture, notably the marked involvement of the anal glands. These are modified sebaceous glands and are regarded as an important excretory organ in skin cases. The use of Silica, Phosphorus, Aconite and Sulphur based on narrow prescribing indications, plus the failure of the Arsenicum to completely resolve the situation, clearly indicated that the core of the condition was not being addressed. Hence the successful introduction of the Dysentery Co. Arsenicum Alb. had been the most successful of the remedies used and it is one of the leading remedies of the associated group. It should be noted that none of the intermittent remedies used with only temporary effect are associated remedies of Dysentery Co, the closest connection being Silica as the chronic of Pulsatilla.

CASE 6.2   A shaky start to a career

A talented but unconfident new veterinary surgeon falls victim to a winter epidemic and fails to throw off its lingering effects until a suitable bowel nosode is administered.

A twenty-five-year-old new veterinary graduate obtained her first position in a companion animal veterinary practice in spite of confessing at the interview that she was extremely nervous and unconfident about actually putting her hard won knowledge into practice. At the interview her subsequent employers had felt that, as she more than adequately filled all other requirements for the job, her self doubts would soon disappear as she settled in. However, in the event, this did not happen, and she continued to require more support than had been anticipated. The clients liked her and her work was good, but even after several months she did not seem to have increased in confidence to any significant degree. It became clear that the problem, rather than a straight lack of confidence, was that she was conscientious to a fault, always asking herself 'have I done every necessary investigation? Have I used the ideal antibiotic?' and other similar questions. She never trusted that a cure was genuine, and agonised over every failure.

After about six months she fell victim to a local epidemic infection, grouped under the non specific diagnosis of 'the flu', and was off work as a result. True to character, she returned to work after three days and subsequently relapsed, then being off work for two further weeks. Her doctor had prescribed a course of antibiotics and various palliative agents without marked benefit. Various other members of the practice had been affected by the illness and Gelsemium 30c had appeared to be helpful, all returning to work quickly. A visit to the young vet after a week established that her symptoms fitted the syndrome of aching muscles, weakness, fever and sore throat typical of the Gelsemium picture, and she was induced to take a 30c night and morning for three days. Her improvement began from that time.

On her returning to work it was clear that she was not her old self. She tired easily, and was plagued by an intermittent low grade sore throat. Any particularly trying or worrying day would trigger a headache. From being a pleasant person who was easy to work with she became easily irritated and sullen.

She had not been involved in the complementary side of the practice, and was tolerant if conventionally sceptical of its activities. She was doubtful as to whether the Gelsemium had assisted her improvement rather than the natural course of the disease, which was, of course, in many ways a legitimate view. That view was reinforced when, after ten days, a further three doses of Gelsemium 30c, night and morning, failed to have any effect. She returned to her doctor who prescribed further antibiotics but these did not improve the situation further. Investigations proved negative for systemic organ disease, including thyroid, and Chronic Fatigue Syndrome. More antibiotics were prescribed, which she finally stopped taking due to their lack of effect. She confided that her bowels had been upset ever since the original illness with flatulence and looseness, and she felt that the antibiotics might be aggravating that.

Increasingly she was becoming depressed by the ongoing situation and finally agreed to give homeopathy another try. Dysentery Co. 30c night and morning for three doses was given. Within forty-eight hours she began to feel brighter, although her bowels had returned to an acute state of diarrhoea. This settled and the flatulence disappeared, although some looseness remained. She continued to improve for a further three weeks by which time she estimated she was sixty percent better but there was being no more improvement. After a month of this stability a further three doses of Dysentery Co. 30c night and morning were taken. The smooth improvement recommenced and after another month she was completely restored. Whether it was the result of her growing experience or the influence of the remedy, she had also acquired an increased confidence in her work. There were no further problems over the next year at which time she left the practice.

Discussion

In spite of the views of the patient, there was no doubt that Gelsemium was the 'genus epidemicus' of the original infection. She was the member of the practice most affected and a number of factors could have contributed to that. Firstly, Gelsemium was taken by the others at an earlier stage of the disease, and it is likely that the stress of the job that the patient was experiencing, albeit self inflicted, had increased her susceptibility. In addition, from the way that the case developed, it would appear that her basic character traits were indicative of a deeper intrinsic susceptibility, and until that aspect was addressed there was no final cure. Gelsemium appears in the amended associated list of Dysentery Co. (see Appendix). The prescription of Dysentery Co. can be regarded on two levels. There was the aetiology of 'Never well since', with the nosode deepening and broadening the action of an associated remedy. Additionally there was the mental dimension with the representation of certain clear character traits of the patient in the remedy picture of Dysentery Co.

CASE 6.3   A young life ruled by fear

Homeopathic treatment is sought for a young dog whose fears are making life difficult for both her and her owner. The prescription of a bowel nosode produces not only an overall improvement but indicates also the remedies required to resolve the problem.

A fourteen month old unneutered Italian Spinone bitch had lived in the same home with a single lady all her life, having come from the breeder at eleven weeks of age. She had been one of a litter of eight and had been the last to leave the breeder. Her present owner had a strong suspicion, based on remarks made by the breeder at the time, that when the last of the other pups had left at around nine weeks old the mother had been removed also leaving the last pup with no company for the last two weeks of its time with her breeder. The present owner had felt that the pup was a little wary and unsure of herself from the outset but thought that time would solve that. Unfortunately the opposite had happened and the growing pup had become more rather than less nervous. By the time of the homeopathic consultation, the dog's fears were dominating both the owner's and her lives: she could not be left at all without considerable distress and continuous barking, and her fear of anything or anybody that she met whilst outside made it impossible to take her for a normal walk. There was never any sign of aggression just frank fear of everything, and any other dog she met produced an exaggerated submissive reaction. Even in her own home she appeared to be on edge at all times and to relax only when all was quiet and the owner quite still. There was a marked fear of fireworks and thunder. There was no urinary or faecal incontinence linked to the fear. Conventional advice had been sought and pheromones had been prescribed without success. The only other suggestion had been tranquilizers and the use of an animal behaviourist, the former being rejected and the latter accepted; consequently an acclimatisation programme was in place but without any marked beneficial after two months. The owner's summary of the situation was that 'stress stops her doing everything'. On her own initiative the owner had tried the Bach Flower preparations Rescue Remedy and Mimulus, as well as a herbal preparation of Skullcap and Valeriana, all without any noticeable effect.

Physically the dog had developed well. She had been fully vaccinated at thirteen and fifteen weeks old, with difficulty because of her nervousness. Her appetite was described as greedy and she had a liking for dried food. Her thirst was 'normal' and she would drink well after eating but infrequently otherwise. Her first season (oestrus) had occurred at nine months old; there had been very little bleeding and her nipples and vulva had swollen noticeably and taken a while to settle back to normal. The owner had noticed a fishy smell from her anal glands occasionally but as there had been no apparent clinical problem no treatment had been given and the situation had resolved on its own. The only other significant event in the history was an enteritis following the first season, with campylobacter being identified as the causative agent. This producing a yellow diarrhoea with blood and mucus; it was treated conventionally and resolved.

A thorough physical examination proved impossible without seriously distressing the dog so the attempt was abandoned. Throughout the consultation (in the dog's own home) the dog was extremely apprehensive, avoiding all eye contact and retreating from the room at the slightest attempt to approach it or even look at it. It was impossible to obtain any further information or form any accurate idea of the dog's temperament or character beyond the continuous fear.

Dysentery Co 30c was prescribed, to be given night and morning for four days. Three weeks later the owner reported that the dog was sleeping more and that friends had remarked that she seemed slightly calmer; the owner was not sure about that but did say that the dog's eyes 'seemed kinder'. The Dysentery Co was repeated night and morning for another four days, this time at 200c. After another month there had been a definite improvement. The second season had just started and a full booster vaccination had been administered without too much difficulty and apparently without adverse effect. The dog was now happier to go out for walks and appeared to enjoy those to some extent, although still nervous. One feature that had developed was a marked fear, for no apparent reason, of two particular corners on one walk and a complete refusal, again for no apparent reason, to go on another route that involved crossing an open field. Behaviour in the home and the separation anxiety had not changed appreciably. The prescription was changed to Arg Nit 200c night and morning for four days. After three weeks her second completely normal season had finished and it was agreed by all her contacts that she was generally calmer and appeared less stressed although still extremely shy, nervous of noise and unable to be left alone. Her three 'terror spots' whilst out were no longer a problem although the difficulties at consultation still continued. The prescription was changed again, this time to Phosphorus 200c night and morning for four days as it was felt that a more phosphorus type of picture was emerging. At the next consultation one month later, again in the dog's own home, there had been a definite improvement; the dog would now approach spontaneously and accept a treat, although any interaction beyond that was still regarded with apprehension. The owner reporting a considerable reduction in the separation anxiety but felt that improvement had ceased. At this point a complication arose in that the dog developed a false pregnancy, producing some milk and becoming extremely protective of and nursing her toys. There was complete regression of all progress in relation to the separation anxiety and the dog became even more attached to her owner than before. Pulsatilla 30c night and morning for four days was administered and over the next ten days the false pregnancy syndrome settled completely, although the separation anxiety did not return completely to its previous improved state. Phosphorus 1M night and morning for three days was prescribed and the improvement was resumed. Further doses at 1M and 10M over the next three months resulted in a dog who, although still of a slightly nervous disposition, was considered to be 'within normal limits'. A final dose of Dysentery Co 1M night and morning for three doses had no further beneficial effect. The owner was unwilling to risk a repeat of the false pregnancy and opted for surgical neutering, which was carried out: recovery was uneventful with no adverse effects on the temperament.

Discussion

In view of the possible aetiology of separation, remedies such as Ignatia, Nat Mur and Chocolate were considered but in view of the uncertainty surrounding the separation and the subsequent presenting picture this approach was rejected. The initial prescription of Dysentery Co was based on the overriding fear being exhibited, which overrode all other approaches, and the theme of 'anticipatory anxiety' associated with the bowel nosode. The increase in potency was decided on following the possible marginal improvement from the 30c dose, and perhaps 200c would have been a more appropriate potency from the start. The change to Arg Nit was on the basis of the three marked and inexplicable fear reactions whilst walking, such reactions being part of the remedy's picture in animals, and the subsequent improvement justified that decision. By this time a clearer phosphorus picture was emerging and so the prescription was changed again with gratifying results.

The prescription of the bowel nosode not only addressed the underlying state in this case but highlighted particular aspects that more local prescriptions were able to deal with although Phosphorus is probably this dog's constitutional remedy. The appearance of the false pregnancy with its accompanying regression of the mental symptoms was treated with, in effect, an acute prescription and did not alter the emerging picture in the long term; in addition the lack of further effect from the final doses of the bowel nosode would support the view of Phosphorus as the correct constitutional remedy. (False pregnancy in the canine is not a true pathological condition but represents a physiological adjustment to an oestrus not followed by a pregnancy) The remedies employed in this case are all associated remedies of Dysentery Co. (see Appendix). Arg. Nit. and Pulsatilla are present in the traditional list but the presence of Phosphorus in the expanded list emphasises the nervous insecurity present in the phosphorus picture.

7

PROTEUS

Traditionally associated remedies
Acid Mur, Ammonium Mur, Aurum Mur, Apis Mel, Baryta Mur, Borax, Calc Mur, Conium Mac, Cuprum Met, Ferrum Mur, Ignatia Amara, Kali Mur, Mag Mur, **Natrum Mur**, Secale Corn.

General considerations

Proteus is a bowel nosode that finds regular application in the clinical situation. It accounted for 3.73% of John Paterson's samples and 3.94% of Elizabeth Paterson's cases. Dogs produced 2.87% and cats 1.85% in the animal survey. The number of swabs in the latter was considerably smaller than in either of the human investigations but it is interesting to note that although the percentage of positive results from dogs was approaching the human levels, that of cats was noticeably lower – in spite of the fact that Natrum Mur., the leading remedy of the associated group, is widely considered to be the archetypal constitutional type for cats! (This is, however, to misinterpret the true nature of the cat's perceived solitary nature, which in the majority of cases it is linked more to its natural social order rather than to any feelings of hurt. In fact all major constitutional types are seen in cats). Although, like Dysentery Co, there are themes of stress and anxiety in the nosode, the nature of these in Proteus is very different. In addition sudden onset, violent outbursts of anger and spasms of both striated and unstriated muscles run through the picture. The major miasmatic influences are psora and sycosis.

In contrast with Dysentery Co, the anxiety and tension engendered in the Proteus type is external in origin, resulting from long periods of stress not of the patient's making. Mention has been made (Chapter 2) of the predominance of chlorine in the associated remedies of the nosode. John Paterson considered that it was the effect of stress on the chlorine metabolism of the body, thereby affecting the balance of the sodium and the chlorine between the cells and the intracellular fluid that was responsible for the 'brain-storm' aspect of the Proteus picture. The adrenal glands are affected by the prolonged stress with the Proteus aetiology and others have suggested a link between those glands and the kidneys via the control of chlorine excretion in the urine (Mount 1973).

Bach considered that the highly strung nervous person with a permanently anxious expression was of the Proteus type, but equally the person with strong emotional control of anxiety as exhibited in the traditional British 'stiff upper lip' is seen just as often. In these cases, when control snaps the result is a sudden outburst of symptoms, either mental and/or physical, with no prior warning. The apparent sudden onset duodenal ulcer, where there are no obvious prior symptoms to suggest its presence (cf. Dysentery Co. Chapter 5), fits this picture, and migraine can arise from the same reaction. In both expressions of the type the attitude attributed to Natrum Mur., the associated group's leading remedy, of 'the triumph of experience over hope' reflects the underlying mental state.

Both of the Patersons found a higher level of marital breakdown, with separation and divorce, among their Proteus patients than in other groups. In view of the times when they were working they considered that the prolonged stress engendered by the Second World War and the time immediately following contributed further to the numbers of Proteus indications found (Paterson 1949). Similar prolonged stress can be engendered in high performance competitive animals as well as in those living in emotionally unsettled environments. Both Ménière's and Raynaud's diseases, with their connections to the circulation and its associated unstriated muscle, are indications for the nosode.

The themes of the nosode, with its nervous involvement and the sudden onset, make it a major remedy for use in epilepsy (Paterson 1949; Saxton and Gregory 2005). Ignatia, one of the associated remedies, is regarded by some as the most commonly indicated remedy in epilepsy (Gregory 2000). Although it is a widely recognised remedy for grief and bereavement, the ill effects of prolonged worry, muscular spasms and sudden onset are also in the Ignatia picture and fit the Proteus symptoms as well. In view of the chemical connection of the Proteus group of remedies, it is also interesting to note that one of the factors linked by some to the successful dietary control of epilepsy is consistency in the intake of chlorine (Carr 2007).

Allergic conditions involving the digestive tract are another indication for Proteus. These represent the genuine allergic reactions with a sudden systemic involvement rather that the dietary hypersensitivities that produce only local symptoms of indigestion and looseness of the motions.

Materia medica

Stress, anxiety and tension are prominent features of the mental state, and a degree of mental instability is part of the picture. There are feelings of being stretched to the limit, until the point when things snap, producing the typical 'brainstorm' with its sudden onset and nervous involvement that are the nosode's theme. This may take the form either of a violent physical outburst or more of an emotional hysteria. Animals may bite, scratch or kick without warning. Children will scream, shout and strike out uncontrollably when angry. Physical cramps and spasms are a common feature of many conditions. The anxiety felt causes irritability and depression with a definite dislike of change. The type has generally closed itself to outside contacts and as a result appears somewhat unresponsive, bordering on antisocial, on many occasions. Feelings of being a victim can easily dominate their thought patterns. However, even whilst they ignore other people, they dislike being ignored themselves and can experience great offence and hurt if they are – they are sensitive to criticism and all too easily feelings of being a victim can dominate their thought patterns. There is a tendency towards fixed ideas and attitudes. Contradiction can produce great anger although there is a liking for consolation.

Frontal headaches are present, with feelings of great intracranial pressure and heaviness. These have a tendency to appear in the week before the menses. The headaches may develop into full migraine with blurring of the vision, vertigo and flashing lights in the eyes. There is a general modality of things being worse in the morning which is seen clearly in the above symptoms, and there may be an accompanying diarrhoea and furring of the tongue. In the author's experience symptoms described for the tongue such as furring and mapping are less reliable in animals than in humans, although they must not be ignored completely.

In addition to the upsets to vision associated with the migraines, the eyes produce acute burning pains that are better for pressure. The eyes are extremely sensitive to light at all times. Meibomian cysts are found.

The digestive system is affected by the general nervous state with a consequent effect on its circulation, leading to constriction of the capillaries. It is this that produces the type of duodenal ulcer that is essentially symptomless until it ruptures, when the first sign is either vomiting of blood or malaena with no prior indication of long-term digestive problems. Ulcers are also seen in the mouth. Such digestive signs as there are involve stomach acidity and associated heartburn. There is pain in the stomach as if from hunger, but eating does not relieve it. Flatulence occurs in both stomach and intestines with abdominal pain. Hiccoughs and vomiting after eating are features, both being a spasm reaction typical of the remedy. Nausea is associated with migraine attacks and diarrhoea occurs through emotional upsets.

Constipation has the sensation of a ball in either the abdomen or rectum and is accompanied by non-productive straining. Stools may be soft and yellow, especially in the morning. The nervous tension may trigger irritable bowel syndrome. Bleeding haemorrhoids are painful. Digestive allergies are seen, with systemic involvement. There is a liking for fats and salt and a dislike of pork, vegetables – notably onions and garlic – and chocolate. There are issues around eggs and butter, with either a strong liking or aversion, and eggs may cause an aggravation. Wine tends to upset the system but there is an overall amelioration from drinking whisky.

Cramps are the main feature involving the muscular system, producing numbness, pain and interference with the blood supply to the tissues. Intermittent claudication occurs. The cramps trigger tendon contraction and interference with the function of the extremities, including weakness. Osteo- and rheumatoid- arthritis may be helped, as may muscular spasm linked to spinal injury. General chronic tension in the system leads to the build up of fibrous nodules in the muscles.

The main feature seen in the cardiovascular system is spasm, affecting principally the peripheral circulation. The effects of this are mentioned elsewhere when the relevant system is discussed, but there are some direct consequences on the heart. Emotions cause palpitations and tightness in the chest. Angina pectoris may be helped, although it must be emphasised that the nosode is not a remedy for genuine cardiac infarction but only for those states where there is constriction of the blood vessels due to spasm (Paterson 1953). The circulation shows an inability to respond rapidly to changes in external heat and there is a general aggravation from either extreme of temperature. Poor peripheral circulation produces tingling sensations in the arms, and chilblains occur. Phlebitis is another consequence of the circulation's poor function.

In the respiratory system there is bronchitis with a productive cough and tightness in the chest that is aggravated by cold. Chronic rhinitis with fluid coryza or blockage of the nasal passages. Pharyngitis accompanied by difficulty in speaking (barking or other appropriate sound for the species).

Cystitis, when it occurs, produces cloudy urine that may be foul-smelling. There are intense burning pains in the urethra. Inflammatory conditions of the female genital system are seen with irritation of the external genitalia. Menses are irregular with much blood and many clots.

The theme of 'suddenness' is seen in the skin with acute oedematous swellings; hence photosensitivity and urticaria, especially in the horse, can respond to the remedy. There can be pustular and vesicular eruptions with intense irritation, but the skin is generally dry. There is hair loss from all areas of the body in appropriate species. Redness and erythema are seen with a tendency to eruptions at the mucocutaneous junctions. An aetiology of loss or grief may be at the root of many skin symptoms.

General modalities include aggravation from lying down at night and also on waking in the morning. The type is worse during storms and for exertion. Aggravation is also produced by either extreme of temperature and from changing suddenly from one to the other. There is a general amelioration from resting, being in mountains, stretching and usually from eating.

PROTEUS	
Mind	'Brainstorm'. Feelings of stress. Irritable. Temper with sudden outbursts. Dislike being ignored. Closed personalities tending towards being loners. Depression. Hysteria. > consolation. < contradiction.
Head	Migraine and frontal headaches. Vertigo.
Face	Burning pains in eyes. Eyes sensitive to light. Meibomian cysts. Cracked lips. Mouth ulcers.
Abdomen	Duodenal ulcers. Flatulence. Pain in stomach. Constipation and diarrhoea alternate. Malaena. Vomiting. Digestive allergies. Rectal spasm.
Appetite	Desires salt and fats. Dislikes butter, pork, vegetables, chocolate. < eggs, wine, onions. > whisky.
Cardiovascular	Spasm of peripheral circulation. Angina pectoris. Palpitations and tightness in chest. Phlebitis. Bleeding haemorrhoids.
Urogenital	Cystitis with cloudy urine. Burning in urethra. Irritant genitalia. Irregular menses. Headaches before menses.
Respiratory	Bronchitis. Pharyngitis affecting voice. Coryza or blocking of nasal passages.
Musculoskeletal	Cramps and spasms. Intermittent claudication.
Skin	Oedematous swellings. Pigmentation. Eruptions at mucocutaneous junctions. Excessive perspiration.
Modalities & Generalities	< extremes of temperature, morning, Lying down at night. > Mountains, resting, stretching, eating, whisky. Ménière's disease, Raynaud's disease. A chilly remedy. Suddenness of symptoms.

CASE 7.1   Lovesick and worried

Physical symptoms defy conventional diagnosis, but homeopathy provides both initial relief of symptoms and, via the use of a bowel nosode, the final solution to the condition.

A four-year-old neutered Border Collie bitch was the subject of an emergency callout one Friday evening. She had appeared normal in the morning but had become quieter throughout the day, especially during the latter part of the afternoon. She had refused her food at 6.00p.m. and at around 8.30p.m. had collapsed whilst out in the garden. There had been no loss of consciousness and it appeared that only the rear half of the body was affected. The attending conventional vet found only intense spasm of the lumbar and sacral regions, with both hind legs in tonic extension. There had been no vomiting or diarrhoea, the abdominal muscles had normal tension and there was no pain on abdominal palpation. The purpose of being in the garden had been to pass water, and this had happened, apparently normally, just prior to the collapse. Rectal temperature was normal and mucosal colour was good. The respiratory rate was slightly elevated but the lungs were normal on auscultation. A provisional diagnosis of acute lumbar disc prolapse was made, analgesic and anti-inflammatory treatment given, and the dog admitted to the surgery.

X-ray and neurological examination the next day found no physical cause for the condition. The evening medication had eased the symptoms to a moderate degree but had failed to give complete relief and the dog was still unable to stand, and would make no voluntary effort to do so. She was retained in the surgery for continued observation and medication. Steroids were administered by injection, also without marked benefit. The dog remained conscious but depressed; water was taken in small amounts but there was no interest in food.

The dog had been left in the charge of the owner's partner whilst she attended a weekend seminar. She had left for this on the Friday morning and was due to return home on the Sunday evening. The lady had acquired the dog as a young puppy. Routine worming and vaccination had been carried out since then, with no apparent adverse reactions. It was some four months since the last medication. Neutering had been carried out routinely before the first oestrus, again without obvious ill effect. The partner had appeared on the scene some two years previously. He and the dog had always got on well, although there had never been the close bond between them that existed between the dog and the lady. The dog had never had any previous back problems, or indeed any major health concerns. She was described as being calm and friendly with no major fears apart from becoming somewhat apprehensive and restless if the lady was absent for any appreciable length of time.

The dog remained in the surgery until the following Monday morning when the lady had returned and was able to come and see her. There was an immediate response to her presence with the dog attempting to stand, although without success, as soon as the two came together. However, by the time the case x-rays had been viewed and the case discussed, a period of some twenty to thirty minutes, the dog had managed to get to her feet, albeit somewhat unsteadily. She was discharged with a course of an anti-inflammatory mixture in tablet form (PLT 200mgm), one tablet to be taken night and morning for one week. A telephone call two days later reported that there had been complete recovery and in fact only one of the tablets had been given, that being on the evening of the day the dog went home. Next morning the dog had appeared normal and was eating again.

The lady normally worked part-time from home, and the seminar she had been on was the first of a course connected with her work. The seminars were scheduled at monthly intervals for six more months. One month later, on the Friday of the next seminar, there was a recurrence of the symptoms. The partner immediately gave one of the PLT tablets still in hand, but to no effect. The dog was admitted to the surgery at the partner's request and further conventional treatment produced only limited benefit. On the Saturday morning the conventional vet sought the help of his homeopathic colleagues. In view of the association on both occasions with the lady having gone away, Ignatia 200c was administered night and morning. By the Sunday morning the dog was able to stand and was eating to a small degree, although still appearing depressed. She was given a further dose of Ignatia 200c and discharged back to her usual home, continuing physically normal but depressed until the return of the lady on the Sunday evening, when she immediately brightened again.

As the lady's course still had six more weekends to go, the longer-term problem of the effect of her absences on the dog was addressed. The first approach was to administer Ignatia 200c night and morning on the Thursday before the lady left, continuing with two doses on the Friday of her departure. This prevented a repetition of the physical collapse but had no effect on the inappetence or the depression, which was still marked. The next month the potency was increased to 1M following the same dosage regime, but the effect was the same. Prior to the next weekend absence four doses of Proteus 30c were give, one night and morning on the Tuesday and Wednesday before departure, followed by Ignatia 1M night and morning on the Friday. This regime produced the desired effect and the dog was her normal self for the whole weekend. At the next weekend, only the two doses of Ignatia 1M were given on the Friday, again with success. After that no medication was necessary although Ignatia was on hand if needed. The dog also became generally less concerned about the lady's shorter absences.

Discussion

This case illustrates the benefits of being able to approach a problem from an alternative and functional point of view. The failure to find a physical 'cause' provided a major hurdle for the conventional members of the practice, and although they could see the possible connection between the attacks and the lady's absence, they had no answer to it other than either sedatives or the lady giving up her course (taking the dog with her was impractical). This case happened in the days before the anti-depressant drugs entered the veterinary market, so perhaps today these would also be considered. One colleague remained in denial and suggested that the improvement following the homeopathic remedies was still only coincidence!

In retrospect, the apparent separation grief that triggered the spasms in the back muscles had beneath it a deeper aetiology of fear and tension, in spite of the seeming calmness of the dog under most circumstances. Ignatia is found solely in the list of associated remedies linked to Proteus. In the original lists it is present only in the first degree, but experience indicates that the second degree rating given it in the Appendix is a more accurate assessment of its worth. The purpose of giving the bowel nosode, and its first level of action, was to augment the action of the Ignatia. However, it is clear that the underlying tensions in the dog were in fact acting as an obstacle to cure. The single course of the nosode was sufficient not only to remove that block, but to do it by having a deeper and curative action in its own right. The hysteria that is such a feature of the Ignatia picture manifested in this case as intense and deep muscle spasm. Its sudden onset, and the nervous involvement involved in it are both major themes of Proteus.

CASE 7.2   Overwhelmed by siblings

Problems arise for a growing child that appear as physical, but which are resolved by a bowel nosode addressing the underlying tensions of family life.

An-eleven-year-old boy was the middle child of three in the family. He had a brother four years older than he and a sister two years younger. The parents were both in full-time professional employment and the family was stable and happy. Within the context of normal sibling tensions, the three children got on well and were devoted to each other.

The elder boy was developing a strong sporting trait. His character was essentially extrovert and outside the schoolroom his approach to life was boisterous and non-academic. The daughter was also an extrovert and had a strong interest in drama, which she indulged to both the amusement and frustration of her parents. All her life she had attempted to keep up with her brothers and as a consequence possessed a definite 'tom-boy' aspect to her character. The younger boy, however, whilst appearing to be an extrovert like his siblings, had a more introverted side to his nature, with a marked studious aspect, although by no means a 'loner'. If something interested him he would become completely absorbed in it. His sporting interest was less than that of his brother; in games of soccer he would participate with enthusiasm and lethal intent in equal measure, but would never be the one to instigate an informal game. He had intimated that he was more drawn towards activities such as golf or cricket, in which he felt he could perform primarily as an individual. His temperament was generally equitable, being only genuinely upset if he were interrupted whilst concentrating on something. On these occasions his temper could be both extreme and vicious, albeit short lived.

Some three months prior to homeopathic help being sought, he had developed small blisters all over his chest, arms and back. They erupted quickly, accompanied by localised redness, and were extremely irritant during this acute stage, occasioning much scratching. When ruptured they contained little fluid but were slow to heal, showing no sign of bleeding or becoming infected, and remaining solely as raw areas. In this more chronic phase the irritation was minimal. In all other respects he continued in good health.

Medical opinion produced no definite diagnosis. A dairy sensitivity was suggested, although there had been no previous indications of this. He drank milk and liked butter, but disliked cheese. Removal of dairy products from the diet, together with local soothing applications had no effect on the condition, and the normal diet was restored. A steroid cream was then prescribed, which relieved the irritation temporarily where it was applied, but had no beneficial effect on the overall condition. The area affected made widespread application both difficult and unpopular and this was soon discontinued. At this stage homeopathic help was sought.

The boy was well nourished and at the time was growing fast. A similar growth spurt some two years earlier had been accompanied by growing pains in the legs, which had responded well to Calc Phos. 30c and there had been no re-occurrence of these. His appetite was good but not greedy. He was not keen on vegetables but this was put down to nothing more than normal childhood dislike. He had a marked aversion to salt, and would not even eat chips if any had been added. There were no other dietary considerations, the only other alimentary feature being a consistent need to pass a motion as soon as he woke, and to pass several motions during breakfast, although the motions were always normal. This trait was not seen at any other meal. Thirst was described as 'average' and urination had never given any problems. He disliked very hot weather and stuffy atmospheres, and would perspire profusely in these situations. Otherwise he appeared indifferent to the climate, and was not upset by reasonable heat in the house. Physical activity did not seem to affect the skin in any way, and there was no excess heat linked to the condition. He had suffered mildly with chickenpox when younger but apart from the usual childhood colds and the pains mentioned above there was no significant medical history. The parents could think of no major event in their lives just prior to the onset of the problem.

Treatment was begun with Sulphur 30c, night and morning for three days. This was selected on the basis of the redness without heat that accompanied the eruption of the lesions, the general reaction to heat and the unusual connection between breakfast and passing motions; this was interpreted as an example of the early morning frequency seen in Sulphur. This treatment, however, produced no change in the condition after 10 days. The parents then volunteered the information that, on reflection, they felt that his temper tantrums 'might have become slightly more frequent', and that six months previously the daughter had started attending a drama class, which had accentuated her natural tendency in that direction.

The prescription was now changed to Staphysagria 200c night and morning for three doses. This was done based on experience with animals, notably cats, where on occasion the slightest change in the group dynamic can trigger skin lesions. Staphisagria has significant skin symptoms and it was thought that the increasing histrionics of his sister may have upset the patient's emotional balance at a deep level, manifesting as skin symptoms, as happens in other species. The essentially easy-going nature of the child coupled with the outbursts of temper were considered to support this approach. This treatment produced an almost immediate improvement in the skin, estimated at sixty percent after two weeks. It was decided to wait, and there was a further slight improvement. After another 10 days this had ceased, although the improvement was maintained.

At this point the patient physically attacked his sister after what was, obviously to him, a particularly annoying episode. Twenty-four hours later he suffered an outburst of blisters, particularly on his arms. Staphysagria 30c was administered night and morning for three doses, which restored the skin situation almost to its previous state, but did not improve it further. There was an 'armed truce' between brother and sister for about a week but then normal relations appeared to be restored. A single dose of Staphisagria 30c at this time produced no further change. The parents were understandably wary about repeating the Staphysagria at the higher potency and so another approach was sought. Proteus 30c night and morning for three doses was given, as modern experience has associated Staphysagria with that bowel nosode. Over the next month the whole situation continued to improve until all that was left was a few lesions on the arms. A single dose of Proteus 200c resolved the issue finally. No further major tantrums occurred and although the patient began to stand up to both his siblings more, this was always solely verbal, always firm but with no hint of violence. The need for the passage of early morning stools remained, but breakfast was no longer interrupted by it.

Discussion

What the effect of repeating the Staphysagria 200c would have been will never be known, and it may have produced the desired result. It was clear that Staphisagria was still the remedy of choice. However, this was an instance where there was an alternative route open to avoid the risk of another physical fight. Staphysagria appears in the amended remedy list as being associated with Proteus (see Appendix), and this is an instance of a bowel nosode being used to avoid the possibility of repeating an undesirable reaction from a still indicated remedy. The 200c potency of Staphysagria was chosen initially because of the perceived mental aetiology in the case. The subsequent reduction to 30c was dictated by caution, as it was considered that the remedy was still working at a deeper level, and all that was required at that stage was a degree of local reinforcement. The reduction in the temper outbursts as well as the removal of the physical symptoms indicates that the core of the 'dis-ease' was now addressed. The dosage sequence of the bowel nosode followed the more traditional pattern of a rising potency as the case progresses.

Although the increased dramatic activities of sister appeared to be the trigger in this case, it seems likely that some tensions also existed between the two brothers, and these were resolved also by the treatment. In spite of the apparently 'normal' relationship between the children, the degree to which a longer- term stress situation existed in the introverted patient faced continuously by two extrovert companions will remain a matter for conjecture. The success of Proteus would indicate that some such stress had been part of the overall picture.

CASE 7.3   A fit of the nerves or something more?

An epileptic dog is controlled reasonably but not completely by anti-convulsant drugs whilst another negative behavioural trait remains untouched. The use of an appropriate bowel nosode resolves the epilepsy and points the way to solving the other behavioural problem.

Both the owner and the attending veterinary surgeon of a three and a half year old neutered female Old English Sheepdog sought homeopathic help for a case of conventionally diagnosed 'idiopathic epilepsy' accompanied by extreme nervousness at all times. The dog had received full initial vaccinations at eleven and thirteen weeks with booster vaccination at seventeen and thirty months of age, all without apparent ill effect. Routine worming had been carried out periodically and there had been surgical neutering at five months old. There had been no physical health problems until the dog was two years old when she had run head first into a park bench and knocked herself out. She had been unconscious for around two to three minutes but the owner had been able to walk her home, a distance of some five hundred yards. A check up revealed no structural damage although she remained somewhat subdued for around a week with an initially very erratic pulse which returned to normal over that time. All appeared well after that until the first convulsion at around three years of age.

The household consisted of a husband and wife and two dogs, living near the centre of a moderate sized town. The other dog, an eighteen month old neutered female Bearded Collie, was dominated by the younger animal. Although dominant to the other dog the sheepdog was described as being basically friendly, very active and quick moving, but extremely nervous and generally 'living on her nerves': at times she could become panic stricken to the point of hysteria for no apparent reason. She had been like that all her life and the situation had not worsened after her accident. The veterinary surgeon considered that this trait was a contributory factor in the epilepsy whilst the owner was convinced that the extreme general nervousness, which continued in spite of all treatments, was at the root of the problem. Without medication the convulsions occurred at roughly weekly intervals with no consistent pattern. They lasted for approximately one minute and began with sudden collapse, involved tonic spasm of all limbs and much salivation but with no screaming and no urinary or faecal incontinence. Recovery was swift with no period of depression afterwards and no increased hunger.

Normally the dog ate well and quickly but was not greedy; diet was a commercial dog food. Thirst was unremarkable and digestive functions were normal. No abnormalities had been found on blood and urine tests.

Conventional treatment was with phenobarbitone at a dosage of 30mgm night and morning which reduced the incidence of the convulsions to approximately one every two to three weeks, again without pattern. Any higher dosage had a marked and unacceptable depressant effect on the dog. Potassium Bromide had been tried but the results had been unsatisfactory and it had been discontinued.

At this stage no change was made to the conventional medication and the initial homeopathic prescription was for Natrum Sulphuricum 30c night and morning for four days, which produced no discernable effect and the fits continued as before. At this point the remedy was changed to Proteus 30c night and morning for three days. Three weeks later there had been no further convulsions and the owner considered that the dog was 'a bit calmer', although what modest improvement there had been had ceased. However, there had been a change in the dog's environment in that the husband and a friend had started an extensive DIY project in the house involving considerable banging and the use of power tools. When this noise was going on the dog lost all semblance of calmness and its only desire was to escape. The other dog remained indifferent to the domestic upset. The Proteus was repeated at 200c night and morning for three doses. This resulted in some definite changes, firstly after eight days the dog was undoubtedly much calmer generally, and secondly she exhibited signs of excessive nervousness only when there was any noise, to which she had become markedly hypersensitive whatever its source. She was still active and there had been no further convulsions.

Theridion 200c night and morning for four days was administered at this stage. Two and a half weeks later the owner reported that the dog was now 'supervising' the DIY work and that it was only a very loud noise that produced any nervous reaction. No further prescription was made and one month later all was still well. The owner was keen to cease the phenobarbitone medication and the dog was weaned off it completely over the next six weeks with no sign of any convulsions. The owner kept Theridion 200c by her and administered a single dose on two separate occasions over the next four months when she felt that the sensitivity might be returning. Nothing further was required and the dog remained calm and free of convulsions. No more booster vaccinations were given.

Discussion

The possibility of a 'Never well since' aetiology involving the head trauma had to be considered, hence the initial prescription of Nat. Sulph. which was preferred to Arnica: Opium and Helleborus were not considered in view of the time interval since the injury. The fact of a booster vaccination after that injury may have had some connection to the onset of the convulsions although there had never been any apparent reaction to any vaccinations and in the event this possible approach was not pursued.

The prescription of Proteus was made on the basis of the close general similarity of epileptic attacks to the theme of the nosode. At first sight the dog's temperament might be thought to resemble the Dysentery Co. type more closely than the Proteus, and hence the selection of Proteus could be considered to have been an 'acute' prescription. However, the themes of the individual nosodes represent fundamental aspects of their pictures (perhaps approaching the idea of the 'essence' of a remedy) and a prescription based on a particular nosode's theme will have a broad based action in a case. In fact the tendency to panic and near hysteria in the dog could be viewed as a form of the 'brainstorm' described in the Proteus theme. The increase in potency of the second prescription of Proteus was guided partly by the start of the DIY and partly by general prescribing principles.

The appearance of a changed and clearer remedy picture is seen frequently after the administration of a bowel nosode, and in this instance the Proteus highlighted the sensitivity to noise which led to a prescription to take the case forward as well as relieving the convulsions. Theridion is not recognised as an associated remedy in the Proteus group but further experience may establish it as such.

8

SYCOTIC CO.

Traditionally associated remedies
Acid Nit, Antimonium Tart, Bacillinum, Calcium Metal*, Ferrum Met,
Natrum Sulph, Rhus Tox, *Thuja Occ.*

*It is unclear what is meant by this entry in Paterson's list but it is included for completeness.

General considerations

Sycotic Co. was linked closely by John Paterson with the sycotic miasm. He
found it represented in 0.32% of his faecal samples, whilst for Elizabeth
Paterson (1960) in her review of cases it represented 16.06% of her total
findings, second only to the Morgan group. In the small animal survey
carried out (Saxton 1994) the figures were 0.57% for dogs and 1.85% for
cats. Although no definite conclusions can be drawn, it is interesting to
consider the relative dates of the three reports. John Paterson based his
survey on swabs taken prior to 1936, the year in which he published his
findings. The cases quoted by Elizabeth Paterson were taken from her
clinical practice in the later years of the 1950s. The animal survey was
conducted between 1991 and 1993. The great watershed within that time
scale was the Second World War, followed by the subsequent expansion of
the chemical therapeutic revolution. Many of the chronic conditions that
are currently seen, and which are apparently increasing, contain a significant sycotic influence due to the suppressive nature of many modern
conventional procedures (Saxton 2006). Thus it may be that the use of
Sycotic Co. will increase accordingly.

The bacteria that form the basis of the nosode were defined by John
Paterson (1933) as diplococcal organisms from the bowels, characterised by
the inability to ferment lactose and also by a failure to react to any of the
other four sugars utilised in the identification of the NLFB. Identification
was by microscopy rather than by culture. He used the term 'sycoccus' to
denote them. It should be noted that these bowel organisms are related

closely to diplococci found in other systems of the body, such as the meningococcus, the pneumococcus and the gonococcus and these reflect the dysbiosis present in those systems such as the respiratory and genital when clinical signs of disease are present in them.

The clinical conditions that are seen in connection with the diplococci involve catarrh to a large degree, and this applies in both acute and chronic conditions. Hence it is not surprising that the bowel nosode finds acute indications in those conditions characterised by the production of catarrh, such as influenza, cat flu, foul pest (Newcastle Disease) and canine distemper. Brown (1967) quotes John Paterson as considering that foot-and-mouth disease in ruminants would be an appropriate use and cites a case of its successful prophylactic use on a farm in Ayrshire. It must, however, be noted that under current UK and EU regulations foot-and-mouth disease is a notifiable disease and its treatment or prevention by private individuals is prohibited by law. Although the connection of the sycotic miasm with gonorrhoea itself is not as straightforward as is sometimes thought, never the less the clinical condition represents a further indication for the nosode.

Sycotic Co. thus finds significant application in acute situations but it is, in common with the other bowel nosodes, in chronic disease that it has its greatest use. Infections are a strong aetiology for its use.

It is instructive to note the remedies used by John Paterson in the treatment of the twenty-two cases on which he based his initial description of the materia medica of Sycotic Co. (Paterson 1932). Only one, Thuja, is in the basic list of associated remedies of Sycotic Co. that is generally accepted today. The others were Medorrhinum, Calc Carb., Drosera, Sepia, Secale, Lycopodium, Hepar Sulph., Nat Mur., Causticum, Tuberculinum and Kali Bich. The majority of these remedies are to be found also in the combined lists of Morgan Pure and Morgan Gaertner that make up Morgan Bach, and this emphasises the importance of the sycotic influence in that nosode in contrast to its commonly perceived solely psoric orientation. Although not included in the list of associated remedies, Lycopodium should be thought of as a complementary remedy to Sycotic Co. John Paterson considered Sycotic Co. to be linked to the tubercular miasm.

The theme of Sycotic Co. is 'irritability', and this applies to both the mental and physical spheres. Mentally this shows as a tendency to sudden outbursts of temper. On the physical level it is the mucous membranes that are primarily affected, especially those of the urogenital system, including a marked involvement of the kidneys. The production of catarrh is a feature. The close link that exists between the sycotic miasm and the urogenital system (Saxton 2006) finds its expression in the inflammatory conditions of the bladder, urethra, uterus and vagina which are strong indications for Sycotic Co. Rheumatic and arthritic conditions are indications for the nosode that are often overlooked.

Materia medica

There is in general a great sensitivity to cold and a general modality of being worse for damp, cold and changes of weather. Initial movement also aggravates. Conditions are improved by heat, prolonged movement and being near the sea.

The irritability associated with the nosode shows itself in the mental sphere as both a general peevishness and outbursts of frank temper. These may progress to hysteria and convulsions accompanied by muscle twitching. There is a nervous restlessness with shyness and a tendency towards depression. A common cause of the temper tantrums is a feeling of resentment. Fears feature prominently, especially of the dark, of being left alone and of animals. However, the tendency to want to hide feelings and weaknesses that is found in the sycotic miasm means that in Sycotic Co. the fears, which may be marked, are often suppressed and patients may appear somewhat withdrawn and uncommunicative. One result of this attempted hiding of what are perceived as negative emotions is the development of behavioural habits as a 'release' mechanism – nail biting is one such pattern that is commonly observed. Headaches may also be triggered by the tensions, being centred in the frontal region, and accompanied by vertigo. They may last for a considerable time, sometimes over several days. Menstruation and sinusitis will also induce headaches in the type. Acute symptoms may resemble meningitis.

Sleep is often restless and unrefreshing with many unpleasant dreams, often involving dead bodies. There is a tendency to grind the teeth during sleep. Patients will either wake early (2a.m.) or be unable to get to sleep until late (3a.m.).

The irritation of the appropriate mucus membranes results in catarrhal discharges from the ears, nose and eyes. Deafness and excessive wax formation are seen in the ears, whilst conjunctivitis, photophobia and tarsal cysts feature in the eyes. There are nasal polyps linked to catarrhal discharges. Ulceration of the membranes of the mouth is also seen. The head shows marked sweating at night, particularly between midnight and 4a.m.

There is difficulty getting to sleep, but this is not usually associated with mental activity. Its quality is generally poor and restless, with nightmares and dreams of dead bodies.

The irritation of mucous membranes produces, in the digestive system, an urgency to pass loose foul-smelling motions, especially in the morning on first rising and immediately after eating. The whole of the tract is affected with distension of the abdomen. There is nausea with burning pains in the stomach, flatulence and vomiting. Constipation is not often seen in relation to Sycotic Co. Gastroenteritis is a common finding, especially in children, with sharp splinter-like pains in the rectum. In John Paterson's twenty-two cases on which the remedy picture is based there were six cases in children under one year of age, and the diagnosis in every case was 'enteritis'. The motion was loose and offensive, accompanied with wasting and anaemia. There are liquid motions after every meal with the diarrhoea being accompanied by sharp pains in the rectum. Some cases show the modality of being better for lying on the stomach. There may be either a desire or aversion for milk, salt and fats; a definite desire for sweets is present plus aversion to vegetables (especially potatoes), vinegar, tea and tomatoes. Eggs produce vomiting and there are digestive aggravations from onions and oranges. Appetite can vary greatly between individuals, but in general it tends towards the indifferent and capricious. There is, however, a definite lack of interest in breakfast and the smell of cooking induces nausea.

There is an affinity for the respiratory system with inflammatory and catarrhal conditions being seen, including acute bronchitis, tracheitis, pleurisy and bronchopneumonia. Pain in the chest wall usually accompanies conditions. Asthma is better when at the seaside but worse for damp and cold. There may be a connection to allergy and hay fever can be linked, especially when of adult origin. The cough tends to be spasmodic and is often difficult to clear. It is worse at night, causing the patient to wake between 2–3a.m. (The use of Drosera quoted in John Paterson's cases involved the treatment of such a cough.) Another feature of the cough is the thick sputum that accompanies it and although expectoration is generally easy it may induce vomiting due to the violence of the coughing. There is chronic enlargement of the tonsils and adenoids with thick mucus production in the throat, and associated lymph node enlargement.

Sycotic Co. has some strong symptoms associated with both the functional and anatomical aspects of reproduction. Although the discharge of leucorrhoea tends to be bland, the discharges from the genital system generally have the copious quantity and fishy smell characteristic of the sycotic miasm. All possible functional upsets of the menses are seen. The irritation of the mucous membranes leads to intense pruritis of the parts, and pain is felt in the left ovary. Vaginal warts, uterine polyps and ovarian cysts occur. Painful inflammatory conditions of the whole urinary system are met with and balanitis is seen in the male. Cystitis and urethritis occur with both urgency and frequency and are accompanied by a strong-smelling corrosive urine containing albumin. Idiopathic sterile cystitis in cats will often respond.

The muscular system is susceptible to fibrositis of the neck, shoulders and back, rheumatism in the arms with nodular deformities of the fingers, and generalised stiffness. However, the more typical rheumatism affects the lower limbs with pain, swelling and discomfort in the feet, accompanied by pain in the knees and loins on walking, and involvement of the sciatic nerve. Pain in the pelvic region is marked on first movement, especially after sitting, although sitting itself is pain-free. In the skeletal system exostoses are seen.

The skin shows greasiness, warts, brittle painful nails and cracks on both hands and feet and around the lips. The warts may be of various appearances but are often large and flat and occur in all locations. All skin eruptions can occur in any location and intertigo is seen and infections in the skin may be found. Skin eruptions can be triggered by vaccination.

A condition associated with the nosode is anaemia, and Kent makes special mention of pernicious anaemia being especially related to sycosis (Paterson 1933). The general connection of the sycotic miasm with new growth is reflected in a tendency towards neoplasia, particularly of the benign type, but malignancies are also seen.

SYCOTIC CO.	
Mind	Irritable with outbursts of temper. Peevish. Restless. Shy. Depression and resentment. Fear of dark, being alone, animals. Hiding of fears and perceived weaknesses.
Head	Frontal headaches with vertigo. Sinusitis. Excessive sweating at night.
Face	Twitches. Facial hair in females. Tarsal cysts in eyes. Photophobia. Wax formation in ears. Catarrhal discharges from nose, ears and eyes. Ulceration in mouth.
Abdomen	Chronic inflammation. Nausea, flatulence and vomiting. Gastroenteritis. Foul-smelling diarrhoea with urgency. Rectal prolapse. Diarrhoea after every meal.

SYCOTIC CO. (continued)	
Appetite	Desires sweets. Aversion to potatoes and other vegetables, vinegar, tea and tomatoes. Either desire or aversion for milk, salt and fats. < eggs, onions and oranges. Indifferent appetite. Nausea at smell of food.
Cardiovascular	Anaemia.
Urogenital	Inflammatory states. Copious bland genital discharges. Fishy smell. Functional upsets to reproductive function. Pain in ovaries (L). Pruritis of all parts. Warts and polyps. Cystitis with urgency and corrosive urine.
Respiratory	Inflammatory and catarrhal conditions. Asthma > seaside. Hay fever. Cough with thick sputum < night. Pain in chest. Lymph nodes enlarged.
Musculoskeletal	Fibrositis, rheumatism and arthritis. Pain in pelvis and lower limbs. Exostoses.
Sleep	Restless. Dreams of dead bodies. Difficulty sleeping.
Skin	Warts and cysts. Greasy. Brittle painful nails. Cracks on hands, feet and lips. Eruptions following vaccination.
Modalities & Generalities	< Cold and damp, first movement. A strongly sycotic remedy. May be of help in acute infections. Where there is much mucus.

CASE 8.1 The obvious is not always the complete answer

A vaccinosis is created by inappropriate conventional treatment. Due to the patient's miasmatic balance, this manifests as predominantly sycotic. An appropriate remedy gives some improvement, but it was not until a bowel nosode is prescribed that the miasmatic balance is moved towards psora and a cure obtained.

A three-year-old entire female English Bullterrier, white in colour, was presented with persistent generalised pruritis that had developed when she was one year old. She had come to her home at eight weeks of age and had received a leptospiral vaccination at ten weeks, followed at twelve weeks by standard canine viral vaccinations for distemper, adenovirus, parvovirus and parainfluenza, together with a second dose of leptospira. There had been no observed reaction to these injections. At nineteen weeks a nasal vaccine had been administered against bordetella bronchiseptica (B. bronchiseptica and parainfluenza are implicated in some 75% of cases of kennel cough in dogs.) Ten days later a mucoid vaginal discharge appeared, which did not seem to affect the dog in any way. A swab showed it to be sterile, no treatment was given, and it disappeared in about one week.

At the same time an otitis externa developed, initially in the left ear but rapidly spreading to the right also. Ear drops were prescribed for this (gentamicin and betamethasone) and three weeks later both ears were clear. Two week after that a routine worming was carried out with a broad spectrum prescription wormer. After a further two weeks a lameness was seen on the left front leg. Physical examination revealed a thickening around the elbow region. Rest failed to resolve the situation and an x-ray ten days later led to a diagnosis of 'short ulna syndrome'. The case was referred to a university veterinary college where NSAIDS were prescribed. The lameness cleared, did not return and no thickening of the tissues was apparent at the homeopathic consultation.

Four months later, in May, the dog began to scratch excessively at her abdomen. A diagnosis of 'possible grass allergy dermatitis' was made and treatment with steroids (prednisolone) by oral administration on a decreasing dosage regime was instigated. This afforded only temporary relief and a month later an antihistamine (Piriton) was introduced, with the prednisolone being given additionally as and when the owners felt it necessary. The diagnosis was changed on clinical grounds to 'atopic dermatitis' and over the next four months investigations for allergies were carried out by means of two blood tests. Diet changes were made as a result of the first test but this produced no clinical improvement.

The treatment regime was continued as before with the addition of one course of antibiotics (cephalexin) and the introduction of a medicated shampoo containing chlorhexidine and miconazole (available as Malaseb). The second blood test produced different results to the first (done by the same laboratory) and in the November an autogenous desensitising vaccine was introduced on the basis of those second results. Skin scrapes and fungal cultures all proved negative. The desensitising injections were continued monthly with prednisolone, chlorphenamine and cephalexin being administered as thought necessary, although without great benefit. A third blood test produced inconclusive results and the only change that was made in the treatment was the addition of a monthly flea treatment containing fipronil (available as Frontline) in spite of no fleas having been seen on any of the three dogs in the household. It was at this point that homeopathic help was sought.

There were two other bulldogs in the household, a neutered male and another entire female. The three were not significantly related and neither of the other two dogs had any sign of skin problems. There was no family history. All the dogs got on well together with no obvious hierarchy. The dog was described as being a friendly outgoing animal who would enjoy fuss if it is offered but would not seek it. She had no known fears and was not upset by thunder in spite of one of the others being terrified. There was great curiosity and extremely sensitive hearing. Appetite was greedy and she would eat anything, but was particularly fond of liver, garlic and onions. Thirst was for large quantities of water at one time and the total intake was described as above average. She would drink some milk but was not keen on it, nor upset by it. The steroids had not increased either her thirst or appetite, but there was a definite weight gain when she was on the higher dosages. Motions were normal and there was no undue flatulence. The owners had not given any steroids or antihistamines for about a month prior to the consultation. There was a temporary worsening of the skin after using the Malaseb shampoo but other preparations could be used without aggravation. The owners' impression was that the desensitising injections helped a bit, and the latest had been given two days prior to the consultation.

The dog had only ever had two oestrus cycles: the first was at six months of age and was normal. The second was not until some fourteen months later and was followed by a severe false pregnancy with considerable milk production and mental depression. Another oestrus was imminent if she was cycling normally but there were no signs of one coming. Her vulva had remained enlarged since the first oestrus. Her teats had become pendulous at the same time. The skin problem had cleared completely during the second oestrus and false pregnancy and had recurred once that was over.

The irritation was generalised. The skin showed patches of redness with areas of marked pigmentation. At times the skin became hot with areas of deep red discolouration. There had been no recurrence of the ear problems and the anal glands gave no trouble. There was a slightly musty smell and greasy feel to the skin. The only sores present had been self-inflicted. The dog liked heat and would seek it out but it did not appear to affect the skin in any way.

The owner was advised to stop the desensitising injections, and treatment was begun with Thuja 30c night and morning for four days, the remedy being chosen on the basis of a probable aetiology of vaccination plus the pigmentation and enlarged vulva and teats, the dietary connection with garlic and onions and the initial left-sidedness of the early symptoms. There was a report ten days later to the effect that the dog was scratching less but the skin was still red. The improvement had been steady and the owners were advised to wait another week. The improvement continued for another two days but at the next consultation the skin had regressed back to its initial state. A potency chord of 30c, 200c and 1M was prescribed night and morning for six days. This produced an improvement that lasted for one week, with less scratching and some fading of the redness in the skin. After that week the skin again regressed but not completely back to its original state.

Sycotic Co. 30c night and morning for four days was then prescribed, followed after one week by two days on Thuja 200c night and morning. This produced no obvious change after four weeks, and two days of Sulphur 30c were administered on the indication of the persistent redness in the skin, again with no benefit. At this point a potency chord of Morgan Bach 6c, 30c and 200c was given for five days. Three weeks later there was a significant improvement in the irritation, although the redness appeared the same. The dog was happy in herself. The other change was the development of a marked body odour.

On the basis of this change, Sulphur 30c night and morning for four days was prescribed, resulting in a significant improvement in all symptoms, and was maintained for five weeks. Accordingly the Sulphur in a potency chord of 6c, 30c and 200c was repeated at that stage and this produced complete resolution of the symptoms. Oestrus still occurs irregularly but each one is normal when it appears and there are no false pregnancies.

Discussion

The initial trigger here would appear to have been, not primarily the vaccination, but rather the suppressive treatment of the reaction to it (Saxton

2005). In view of the continuing slight functional abnormality of the reproductive system it is likely that the inherited miasmatic balance in this
animal was predominantly psoric/sycotic. True adverse reactions to vaccination are more commonly seen as a result of vaccines given by injection
rather than the administration of those following the natural route of infection. In this case it would seem that the appearance of the vaginal discharge
and the otitis represented a normal exteriorisation by the body of a challenge, and both the mucoid nature of the discharge and the involvement
of the ears pointed to a sycotic influence. The treatment of the ears, the
development of a lameness with tissue thickening and the apparently
successful use of a NSAID leading on to a manifestation on the skin, all
indicated a suppression of that sycotic influence. The nature of the skin
symptoms also fitted in with sycosis. Thus Thuja was selected as an anti-
sycotic remedy that fitted the presenting symptoms. Its positive but limited
effect, especially after the use of a potency chord, indicated a block to
progress rather than a wrong remedy selection and the use of Sycotic Co.
was designed to address this. However, the failure of both further doses of
Thuja and a course of Sulphur to carry the case forward indicated that
another approach was indicated. Morgan Bach was chosen as covering all
the indicated remedies and this resulted in moving the case towards
Sulphur, with its subsequent successful use. It is interesting to note that the
effect of the Morgan Bach was both to indicate more clearly the need for
Sulphur and to enable it to have its full action.

What the effect of giving Morgan Bach earlier in the case, rather than
Sycotic Co., would have been will never be known but it is possible that its
balance of psora and sycosis would have fitted the case better and given a
swifter resolution.

CASE 8.2   The ravages of time

*An indicated remedy produces some improvement of a palliative nature. An
appropriate bowel nosode is introduced with the aim of augmenting the
remedy's action, but in the event the nosode appears to act as a remedy in
its own right.*

A fourteen-year-old neutered male cat was presented with a general
complaint of 'slowing down'. On questioning this was clarified to a
marked unwillingness to move. Although still bright and alert and
wanting to eat and drink he was no longer interested in going outside,
and spent most of his time in his basket. Appetite had always been

adequate rather than greedy, although what food was taken had always been eaten with enthusiasm. There was now a distinct reluctance to move quickly to his food when it was put down, but once there he ate as well as ever. He remained standing whilst eating and drinking. He had always been fed on commercial foods and was not keen on the dried formulations. His thirst had increased slightly over the last few years but was by no means excessive. The weight was within the normal range for a cat of his size and was stable. He was fully continent and had a litter tray inside that he used infrequently. Motions were normal and a urine sample showed only a slight amount of albumen present on dipstick, with all other parameters being clear. Physical examination revealed no significant abnormalities except for some tenderness on palpation around the pelvis and lower spine. The owners declined the offer of blood tests and x-rays in view of the sedation that would necessary, and a tentative vague diagnosis of a musculoskeletal condition affecting the lower spine was made, with conservative treatment being requested. The owners were against any form of conventional medication and enthusiastic about homeopathy. Hence this was the option agreed on, with the possibility of acupuncture being held in reserve.

The cat had always been the only animal in the house. He was friendly and over the years had been playful. His was essentially a placid temperament but the owners had the impression that he was afraid of some things, although they had never been able to identify them. He had always gone outside readily in all weathers but had always remained close to his own garden. On occasion he had been seen to defend himself vigorously but never to start a fight. He did not resent being examined and made only a half-hearted attempt to move away when the painful areas were palpated. He liked heat and would lie in the sun or near any source of heat. If he did move for any reason he would have a short walk around the ground floor of the house but would not attempt the stairs. The owners could not identify any clear modalities for the condition.

The medical history contained occasional minor injuries, bites and two incidents of non-specific pyrexia, all of which had been treated homeopathically. Routine vaccination had ceased at six years of age and no routine flea treatments had been given. The only significant event had been an injury to the right stifle (knee) some two years previously. A diagnosis of cruciate damage was made on purely clinical grounds and was treated successfully with Ruta Grav. and Gelsemium, both at 30c, over a period of three weeks. There had been no further problems with the leg, and the cat was walking sound on it. The present problem had come on gradually over a period of some months.

Rhus Tox. 30c was administered night and morning for five days. The choice was made rather on general principles, with the liking for heat being extrapolated into a dislike of and possible aggravation from cold, and the only modality straw to clutch at being the fact of the cat going for a short walk after having moved for some imperative. This produced a definite improvement of around 50% (owners' estimate) but it was only maintained for around two days after the end of the course. Although the general vitality of the cat was considered reasonable, an increase of potency to 200c was thought to be inadvisable in view of the age of the cat, the degree of slowing and the implications of that for the strength of the vital force. Accordingly Rhus Tox. 30c was repeated night and morning for two days followed by a single dose every other day. This had the desired effect of maintaining the improvement but there was no significant increase in it, and any cessation of the regime resulted in a rapid deterioration.

After a month of attempted adjustments around this regime without success, the remedy was changed to Sycotic Co. 30c night and morning for four days. This was introduced whilst the improvement was still present, with the result that initially the situation remained stable, and after ten days there were signs of further improvement. This increased to around 80% and remained at that level for six weeks before beginning to regress. A single dose of Sycotic Co. 30c restored the situation. A further two day course of Rhus Tox. 30c night and morning gave no additional benefit. Subsequently the situation was maintained for eighteen months with Sycotic Co. 30c in single doses as necessary until the cat died of natural causes.

Discussion

It was unfortunate that the owners' aversion to medication, even a sedative for diagnostic purposes, meant that all pathological conclusions in this case were inevitably tentative. The Rhus Tox. had produced a definite if limited benefit and the Sycotic Co. was introduced in the hope that it would augment that. In the event it became clear that it was in fact acting as a remedy in its own right. It must, of course, be pure speculation that the cat was experiencing the pains in the lumbar-sacral region and the stifles that are found in the remedy picture, together with the weakness and pains in the legs. At no stage was there any licking or biting at the feet which might have indicated pains in them. The action of the remedy was certainly palliative rather than curative, but it seems probable that physical changes in the spine were producing an insurmountable obstacle to cure.

CASE 8.3 An obstacle to academic achievement

Homeopathic remedies are given, with some success, for a disabling condition. However, it is not until the introduction of the bowel nosode that the desired breakthrough is obtained.

The eighteen-year-old only son of a veterinary surgeon and a general medical practitioner had begun to suffer from sinusitis. All through his life he had been prone to minor upper respiratory problems. As a child he had been susceptible to colds, seemingly triggered by any damp weather conditions, and autumn and winter colds continued to be an ongoing problem. Matters always improved in the summer months although the link to dampness persisted. He had never suffered from Hay Fever. The intensity of individual attacks had varied, from a blocked nose and slight unproductive cough to a bilateral watery nasal discharge with a moist cough and slight respiratory embarrassment on exertion. Occasionally this was accompanied by a sore throat but usually there was no interference with appetite. Usually there was no significant sneezing, with tonsils and cervical glands not being involved. Herbal Echinacea was used regularly plus courses of antibiotics as felt appropriate by the parents. Over the past eighteen months the pattern had gradually changed to attacks more typical of sinusitis. These presented with a blocked feeling in the nose that was not easily relieved by any means, tenderness around the frontal areas of the face, especially on the right side, and bilateral frontal headaches with feelings of pressure. Such nasal discharge as was present at those times was grey in colour, thick and stringy. Between acute attacks an almost continuous watery discharge from the right nostril had developed. At best, courses of antibiotics were giving minimal relief. At their worst the symptoms were interfering with his ability to study and, general health issues apart, increasingly this aspect of the situation was causing concern.

Apart from the respiratory problems, the boy's health had been generally good. He had been vaccinated routinely in childhood. He was not of a sporty disposition but enjoyed walking and swimming if on holiday in sunny climes. His parents described him as 'normally fairly quiet but can be impatient. He can be obstinate and have a violent temper occasionally but basically sociable and friendly.' His appetite and thirst were considered to be unremarkable. He had a strong dislike of curry and garlic. He would take milk happily in tea and coffee or on cereal but would not of choice drink it on its own. He had never tried oysters because he didn't 'fancy the look of them' but had an otherwise catholic taste. If chocolate was available he would tend to gorge himself but was by no means a 'chocoholic'. His digestion was good and he rarely suffered from flatulence or diarrhoea. He liked the open air although not if there was too much wind. He enjoyed heat as well although during his respiratory attacks he disliked too stuffy an atmosphere. He had no marked fear of noise, his dislike of storms being more to do with the rain rather than the thunder. At the time of the initial consultation the latest acute episode was failing to respond to yet another course of antibiotics.

Dulcamara suggested itself because of the link to dampness as a trigger. Natrum Sulph was briefly considered but did not seem to be appropriate in view of the character of the boy. Dulcamara 30c was hence administered night and morning for three days. As a result the pressures around the head eased to a moderate degree and the discharge from the right nostril increased. These changes occurred over about one week and remained stable after that, in spite of repeating the Dulcamara 30, night and morning for three doses after a further two weeks. At this point the remedy was changed to Silica in the hope of stimulating a significant drainage from the nose. The degree of inflammatory reaction that must inevitably have been present in the affected soft tissues was an additional factor in the choice of Silica. A 30c potency was given night and morning for three doses followed by two single doses, one after seven and the other after fourteen days. This had the desired effect and a more copious bilateral nasal discharge of grey, thicker mucus appeared almost immediately, although the feelings of pressure around the head persisted. The discharge continued at the same level for one month from the initial doses of Silica with no signs of ceasing or of further general improvement in the patient.

At this point Sycotic Co. 30c was prescribed night and morning for three doses. After four days the nature of the nasal discharge had changed to a more yellow colour and although still copious had become less stringy. Much of the pressure around the head eased and the patient felt better generally. After about a fortnight the discharge ceased. The patient appeared to be clear in the head but shortly after the thin watery discharge recommenced from both nostrils. A single dose of Sycotic Co. 200c was given. This produced twenty four hours of copious yellow discharge which then ceased spontaneously and there has been no recurrence of the problem. Some two years later the whole family suffered from 'flu' but that resolved without triggering any longer term respiratory problems in the patient.

Discussion

The connection to dampness in this case that suggested Dulcamara as a possible remedy is a feature of the sycotic miasm, with which the remedy Sycotic Co. has a close association. Neither of the two remedies initially used here, both of which produced some effect, feature in the original associated remedy list for Sycotic Co. but both are included in the amended list that modern experience has created (see the Appendix for details). In view of the influence of the sycotic miasm, earlier use of the bowel nosode may have produced a swifter effect, especially in view of the prior use of antibiotics over a considerable period of time. However, a satisfactory outcome was obtained once the underlying imbalance in the case had been addressed by the Sycotic Co. It is interesting to note that, whilst Dulcamara is listed as a leading sycotic remedy, Silica is more generally regarded as tubercular (Banerjea 2003). It might have been expected that a significant tubercular influence in this case would have shown as a Hay fever aspect to the syndrome but in the absence of that it would appear that the case was firmly rooted in the sycotic miasm.

9

GAERTNER BACH

Traditionally associated remedies
Calc Fluor, Calc Hypophos, Calc Phos, Calc Sil, Kali Phos, **Merc Viv**,
Natrum Phos, Natrum Silicofluor, **Phosphorus**, Phytolacca Dec, Pulsatilla
Nig, **Silicea**, Syphilinum, Zinc Phos.

General considerations

Gaertner Bach has the closest link to the syphilitic miasm of all of the bowel
nosodes, and there is also a connection to the cancer miasm. Although
Syphilinum is not listed as a leading remedy of its associated remedy group,
nevertheless John Paterson (1936) stressed its usefulness in cases where the
appropriate NLFB are found in the stool. Wheeler (1924) stressed a psoric
side to the picture, citing Sulphur, Lycopodium and Psorinum as having
connections. John Paterson found the NLFB in 1.27% of his samples whilst
Elizabeth Paterson identified them in 3.33% of her clinical cases. No
positive findings were recorded among the dog and cat samples (see
Chapter 2), although the small size of the samples may account for that.
Certainly Gaertner Bach is as useful in animals as any of the other bowel
nosodes.

The Gaertner NLFB have been found particularly in cases of malignancy
(Roppe, quoted by Agrawal 1995) and the changing patterns of disease,
particularly the increase in the incidence of malignancies in modern times,
may well be leading to an increase in the indications for this nosode. It
must not be thought, however, that its usefulness is limited to such
conditions.

The theme of the remedy is generally regarded as 'malnutrition', which
may arise from a number of causes, and emaciation is a common accom-
paniment to that condition. However, 'emaciation' should be considered
as another theme in its own right, and marked emaciation is itself a strong
indication for the use of the nosode, whatever the cause. Nor should its

use be forgotten in cases where weight and general health have been lost due to an acute condition that has been resolved, but where there is an ongoing failure to thrive in spite of good nutrition and other management/lifestyle factors. The nosode has a strong connection with nutrition in general and its greatest action is seen in the alimentary system, and anything that interferes with the normal digestive and absorption functions of the bowel may produce the remedy state. Such conditions are frequently found at the extremes of life. The nosode is sometimes called the 'children's nosode', and problems at the time of weaning, with the change over from mother's milk to a more solid diet may call for it – indeed any disturbance of the alimentary tract in children may be helped. Elizabeth Paterson recommended its use for teething in cases where other remedies, especially Chamomilla, failed to act. Its use is particularly recommended in cases where teething is linked to recurrent ear problems (Agrawal 1995). In these cases a dose of Gaertner Bach 30c and a dose of Silica 30c the next day is recommended. Fast-growing children on a poor diet can also benefit – indeed any child or young animal that is failing to thrive may be helped.

An aetiology of infection may be present, especially if upsets subsequently occur from the overuse of antibiotics, and the nosode is one of the remedies of use in clearing a case that has been abused in this way. The nosode should be considered in cases of coeliac disease. Digestive allergies, particularly those affecting the colon may also be an indication. It is also of use in cases of worm infestations although, of course, additional appropriate treatment to remove the worms will be necessary. The nosode is claimed to clear threadworms from the body, but in the author's experience it is unwise to rely completely on homeopathy for the elimination of any type of worm.

Malignancy of the bowel, especially in the elderly, is another major indication, where the accompanying emaciation may be the initial sign that is recognised.

Any case of intractable diarrhoea with the almost inevitable loss of condition, whatever the cause, may be helped by the nosode.

Two features that often, but not invariably, accompany these conditions are, firstly that the malnutrition and emaciation occur in spite of a good appetite, and secondly that they are often accompanied by much mental activity, sometimes tipping over into physical hyperactivity.

Materia medica

There is no marked laterality to the nosode. Nervousness, apprehension and cold will aggravate all symptoms. There is an amelioration in company and also from heat, although a stuffy atmosphere will aggravate.

The mental state is marked by much nervous activity and very great sensitivity to stimuli at all levels. Wheeler considered it to be the supreme remedy for neurasthenia (1924). Problems with communication and feelings of vulnerability are seen. High intelligence is seen and children can appear precocious, although depression, irrational guilt and lack of confidence are also found. There may be pessimism and a generally negative attitude to life. Patients can be 'talked out' of these latter but quickly revert if the encouragement is removed. Fears are intense, particularly about the dark and being alone, which may be a reflection of the general lack of confidence that is often seen in the type. There is much brooding and worrying about all aspects of life, sometimes leading to resentment about particular things. Sleep can be restless and accompanied by unpleasant dreams. Children will often need a nightlight on or the company of another person, preferably the mother; although once they are asleep they will sleep for a long time. This insecurity is also seen in anticipatory anxiety when faced with new situations, and these will be avoided wherever possible. When faced with new situations and people, the coping mechanism includes conforming to the group and a desire to please its members. The associated mental unease and insecurity leads to a need to know exactly what is happening, and why, at all times. The sensitivity to noise can be so great that it spills over into fear, and storms are particularly distressing. There are also nameless fears and a tendency to claustrophobia. There is a restlessness about the type, primarily involving the limbs; also an inability to concentrate, and general excitability. Trifling matters upset and irritate them very easily. Children will bite their nails and animals may similarly nibble their feet or lick other local areas of the body.

A range of subjective eye symptoms are a feature, with flashes of light and dark specks being commonly recorded, without corresponding pathology of the eye. Ear discharges, especially in children, are found and idiopathic deafness has been helped on occasion (Wheeler 1924).

The cardiovascular system is similarly affected with either purely subjective symptoms such as palpitations, or, if a lesion is present, symptoms out of all proportion to its severity. Arterial degeneration is also seen.

The mouth has dry eruptions around the lips and fissures on the tongue together with much salivation. The teeth are of poor quality and may be blackened. Gastroenteritis is commonly seen with pain in the stomach, and both mucus and blood in the motions. Excess acidity leads to dilation and discomfort of the stomach. Vomiting occurs easily, especially after sweets, for which there is a strong desire. The vomiting will often induce a headache. There is also a desire for oats, cheese, sugar, eggs and milk puddings, although eggs and milk may upset. Aversion to bread, butter and animal and fish protein is found. The appetite may be faddy, and it is one of the remedies to consider when patients require constant dietary stimulation and changes of food to keep them eating. The most marked feature is an inability to digest fats. Constipation is seen but the more common feature is an offensive diarrhoea with a cyclical pattern accompanied by irritation around the anus.

Colds with a cough that is worse at night are seen, with some involvement of the bronchi. Nasal catarrh accompanies this, and nasal polyps are also found.

The genital system is not a major site of activity for the nosode, the only symptoms being a copious offensive leucorrhoea with pruritis of the genitalia in the female and hydrocele in the male. The urinary system is affected, with blood and mucus in the urine and burning in the urethra.

Rheumatism and fibrositis are seen in the shoulders, hands and feet. Irritant blisters occur on the soles of the feet. Sciatica and great pain in the lower back and hips is described. All the symptoms are worse at night.

Pustular skin eruptions are found on the head, neck and back, together with urticarial eruptions. There is a susceptibility to chilblains, and boils on arms and legs feature in the picture.

GAERTNER BACH	
Mind	Nervous activity. Overactive mind. Great sensitivity to stimuli. Intelligent, precocious children. Pessimism > encouragement. Marked nameless fears. Easily upset. Excitability.
Head	Vomiting induces headache.
Face	Functional disturbances of eyes. Mouth ulcers. Eruptions around lips and tongue. Poor quality teeth. Ear discharges and idiopathic deafness.
Abdomen	Acidity with dilation and pain in stomach. Vomiting especially after sweats. Blood and mucus in motions. Offensive diarrhoea. Inability to digest fats. Allergies.
Appetite	Desires oats, cheese, sugar, eggs and milk puddings. Aversion to bread, butter, animal protein. Capricious and faddy appetite.

GAERTNER BACH (continued)	
Cardiovascular	Palpitations. Arterial degeneration. Severe symptoms.
Urogenital	Copious offensive leucorrhoea. Irritant genitalia. Blood and mucus in urine. Urethral burning. Enuresis.
Respiratory	Nasal catarrh and polyps. Cough < night. Bronchitis.
Musculoskeletal	Sciatica and pain in lower back and hips. Rheumatism and arthritis in shoulder hands and feet.
Sleep	Restless. Unpleasant dreams.
Skin	Eruptions on back, head and neck.
Modalities & Generalities	< cold, nervousness, stuffy atmosphere, night > company, heat. An aetiology of use/overuse of antibiotics. Scratching/biting nails from nervousness.

CASE 9.1 A frustrating dog

An apparently healthy dog is affected by appetite problems and inability to gain or retain body weight. The use of the indicated bowel nosode and some of its associated remedies produces the desired effect.

The frustration in this case was felt by the owner of a fifteen-month-old neutered female boxer dog with an eating and weight problem. The dog had been acquired at eight weeks of age and had appeared normal in all respects. Although she had been the smallest of a litter of six she had been within the acceptable size range for a litter. Whilst still with the breeder she had gained weight steadily in proportion to her size but had not caught up with her litter mates to any significant degree. The first part of the standard vaccination course had been given when she was eight weeks old, immediately after leaving the breeder, and this was followed by the second injection at twelve weeks. A booster vaccination had been given three weeks before the first homeopathic consultation. There had been no observed reactions to these procedures. Routine worming had been carried out by the breeder using a product freely available on general sale, and following that a broad spectrum prescription-only anthelminthic had been administered after the second part of the primary vaccination. Subsequently routine broad spectrum worming had been carried out at approximately four month intervals using prescription products.

The owner was a single lady and there were two other dogs in the household, a Border Collie and a Cocker Spaniel. Although both were older than the patient, neither was an old dog, and as the owner had a large garden with access to woodland, all three got much exercise. They were friendly together and the owner was unable to identify a top dog between them. The only hint of possible trouble came from the patient, who was vocally territorial. Any visitors would set her off into a paroxysm of barking, although once it became clear that they were acceptable and were admitted she ceased, gave them a brief examination and then retired. The other expression of this trait was that if she was in her bed and anyone, either owner or one of the other dogs, came too near she would growl. She had never done more than that and the owner was not worried as she did 'not think that she meant it', since if she was ever shown any aggression by another dog she would immediately run off.

The dog was described as being extremely lively and interested in everything. She liked attention, but would rarely stay still long enough to receive much fussing, although she appeared to like it one the few occasions when it had happened. She was basically obedient and was described as being sensitive to all impressions and moods. She had no great fears, but was worried by noise if she did not know where it was coming from. She was keen on heat and would lie in the sun and near a fire if possible. Continuous exposure to heat did not cause her to pant excessively or become in any way distressed. She was happy to go out in cold weather provided it was to do something active.

Although her skeleton had grown normally, she had always been on the thin side. She was living an extremely active life and had a poor appetite. This combination had been thought to be the cause of the thinness and no action had been taken. She had been neutered at six months of age, before her first oestrus (menses), without any complications. At the physical examination prior to surgery, and also at the check over prior to vaccination, all had appeared normal.

When she was ten months old there had been some weight loss, with no illness or other upset to account for it, and no change in temperament or activity. The owner had tried several changes of diet to correct this but with no great success. There had been some temporary weight gain on a raw meat diet, but this had subsequently been lost again. One of the problems throughout this time had been the dog's unwillingness to eat either well or consistently.

Investigations revealed a slight elevation of the liver enzymes, but these were not considered to be clinically significant. Bile acid and foliate tests were normal, as was enzyme estimation for exocrine pancreatic function. All other blood and urine parameters were within normal values. Physical examination revealed no abnormalities. Motions were normal in appearance and frequency. There was no undue flatulence or signs of abdominal pain after eating.

At the time of the homeopathic consultation her weight was 18.7kg and all her ribs and major bony outlines of the body were clearly visible. Thirst was unremarkable. The dog had always been a poor eater, requiring frequent changes of diet. She would appear keen on one particular food for a few days, eating with apparent enthusiasm, although never in large amounts. Then she would lose interest in that food and stop eating completely until something new was introduced, and the pattern would repeat itself. There was no food for which she showed any marked enthusiasm. Even if the owner managed to keep her eating there was never any significant weight gain. At no time had there been any change in her activity and she appeared as a happy and contented dog.

The initial treatment was with Tuberculinum Bovinum 30c night and morning for four days, the remedy being chosen on its clinical picture. This produced an almost immediate improvement in the dog's appetite, with regard to both the willingness to eat and the quantity taken. However, the improvement had only taken the appetite into the adequate range and although the owner had felt after one week that there had been some weight gain (a subjective assessment based on the visibility of the ribs), after a month the situation was essentially unchanged. The weight on re-examination was 19.1kg. It was felt that some additional stimulus to the system was required at this point and hence Gaertner Bach 30c was added to the treatment, night and morning for three days, followed by a repeat of the Tuberculinum 30c once daily for seven days.

After a further five weeks there had been a slow but steady gain with the weight increasing to 22.5kg. The appetite had not changed. The only other change had been an increased sensitivity to noise and sudden movements. Three weeks later the situation was stable but unchanged. Gaertner Bach 30c was repeated as above and the slow weight gain recommenced. The nosode was repeated after one month, a dose night and morning for one day, and again after a second month. After that time the weight had increased to 26.2kg which was considered adequate in view of the dog's size. No further treatment was given and all continued to be well. There was no significant further gain and the appetite continued to be steady although still only adequate.

Discussion

The root of this problem would appear to lie in a deep-seated congenital imbalance in the function integrity of the metabolism. Although there was not the classic Tuberculinum picture of weight loss in spite of a good appetite in this case, the initial treatment was given on the basis of the activity and curiosity of the dog, plus the feeding characteristic which is a well recognised tubercular pattern in animals. There was obviously some resonance with the remedy in view of the improvement in the appetite, but the failure to gain weight accordingly indicated the need for an additional approach. Tuberculinum is an associated remedy of Gaertner Bach and the nosode was given as a means of enhancing the action of the Tuberculinum, hence the close proximity of the two courses. The change in the dosage regime of the Tuberculinum was made in the hope of the combined effect producing a sustained benefit to the appetite. The subsequent course of the case, with no further increase in the appetite, indicated that it was the Gaertner Bach rather than the Tuberculinum that was addressing the underlying problem. The dosage pattern for this was chosen in view of the slow progress being made. Whilst the vitality of the patient appeared to be high, for some reason this was not being utilised as expected. On general principles, repetition of the same potency was indicated, as some progress was being made and maintained, and it is the author's policy never to increase the potency of an associated remedy when a bowel nosode is introduced. Without the introduction of the Gaertner Bach, an increase of the Tuberculinum to 200c could have been considered. An additional course of Tuberculinum could also have been considered at the end of the treatment, but it was thought unlikely that it would have helped further, and the owner was happy with the outcome.

CASE 9.2   Vital support for a failing system

A geriatric patient is helped in the closing years of his life by the periodic prescription of the relevant bowel nosode.

An eighty-nine-year-old man had lived on his own following the death of his wife some five years previously. Although age had been taking its toll steadily, he had an independent nature, and had fiercely rejected any suggestions of alternative accommodation.

He had been a fit, healthy and active man all his life, with a passion for walking, golf and travel. He distrusted the activities of doctors, based on a conviction, which grew as he became older, that he had only to enter a surgery to be admitted to a hospital, of which places he had a morbid fear. At the same time, paradoxically, he had a blind faith in his doctor's advice on those occasions when he did consult him. Both these attitudes were accentuated by his complete inability to understand medical matters, no matter how much he read or how often things were explained to him. His did, however, attend regularly for his annual 'flu' injection. He had suffered a stroke when eighty-two and following this and routine blood testing in relation to cholesterol, he had been prescribed a statin drug (Simvastatin) prophylactically. In addition he took a range of commercial supplements covering vitamins A, D, E and selenium, which habit had been established by his wife, and to which he still broadly adhered. He had recovered well from the stroke, the only permanent effects being a tendency to fall to the left and a loss of the appreciation of time. His medical history was otherwise sparse. There had been two attacks of cystitis in the six months after his wife died. The first had apparently resolved itself, but the second a few weeks later had been so severe that he was compelled to seek help. The problem had responded to oral antibiotics and not recurred. The loss of his wife had accelerated his general mental decline, particularly with regard to his short-term memory. One consequence of that was that the taking of his routine medication became somewhat erratic.

As his family lived nearby it was possible to keep a close eye on him, and the situation had been manageable until events took a more acute turn.

It had become clear that he was losing a worrying amount of weight. He refused to visit his doctor, maintaining that he 'felt fine'. There was no vomiting, and bowels and bladder were functioning normally. His appetite, as assessed during family meals, was initially good (as it had always been) and his thirst had not increased. He was sleeping more than in the past, but not excessively, and was reasonably bright when awake. His only complaint about his health concerned his failing eyesight. There had been a general deterioration and in addition his optician, who had done all he could with spectacles, had diagnosed mild cataracts in both eyes, although surgery had not been discussed.

It was finally established by the family that he was basically just not eating enough. The food he bought for himself consisted almost entirely of a narrow range of ready-made fish meals from the supermarket, which he admitted to being bored with. Added to that was the increasing difficulty he experienced seeing the controls on his cooker. The result of all this was that, as he admitted, he 'couldn't be bothered' to eat and his appetite had decreased. Meals left for him by his family were not being eaten, partly because of the difficulty of heating them up, and partly because on occasion he just forgot about them. The result had been that he was essentially living on a bowel of cereal every morning, two lunches cooked for him by his cleaning lady during the week and Sunday lunch with his family.

He was encouraged to give more attention to his diet, and a closer general monitoring of him was instigated. Homeopathic treatment was introduced and three doses of Tuberculinum Bovinum 6c were given over twenty-four hours as a constitutional prescription. This was felt to be the remedy of choice given his love of travel and activity in the open air, His purchase of only fish dishes fitted in with his lifelong preference for fish as opposed to meat, with mackerel being his favourite. He had great caution, if not outright fear, towards dogs generally and large dogs in particular – he had been bitten on several occasions without offering any provocation (a case of animals 'smelling' fear?) Possibly his complaint that he had become 'bored' with fish could be considered as another reflection of his Tubercular trait.

There was a general brightening of his demeanour, his food intake improved, and the weight loss stopped. However, he was now receiving closer support and supervision and this may have been the main source of the improvement. Although, with encouragement he was now eating better, his appetite had reduced in size, and there was no weight gain.

Five months later he had suffered a fall, which had severely bruised his chest and pelvic region on the left side. There had been a skin wound on his scalp and he had become more confused mentally, leading to the suspicion that he had hit his head in the fall, possibly on the edge of a small table. There had been no nystagmus or headache. He had been unable to stand as a result of the fall, although medical examination revealed the only bony damage to be two cracked ribs.

He had been admitted to hospital for observation, and it had quickly become clear that the incident had produced a profound effect on his whole body. Both liver and kidney function had been put under stress, although he had not gone into organ failure. Treatment had been conservative, and because of being in the hospital, no homeopathic aid had been given. The pain and bruising had subsided slowly but he had remained mentally depressed and confused as to his whereabouts.

He had been discharged from hospital after one week. Arrangements had been made for him to enter a care home, initially on a convalescent basis. Homeopathic treatment was given, mainly in view of the mental state, and the home was happy for this to be used. Arnica 30c night and morning was administered for three days. This was a pathological prescription based on the bruising and the aetiology of a fall. As the bruising was resolving anyway, it had been difficult to assess the effect of this, but there had been no dramatic change in his mental state. Accordingly, the remedy had been changed to Opium 30c night and morning for three doses, based on the drowsiness and stupor seen in that remedy's picture. Following this his confusion had cleared, although he had been still somewhat slow and non-reactive. The Opium 30c had been repeated at the same dose after three weeks, resulting in him becoming able to be stimulated more easily, although still remaining mentally slow.

At this point the occupancy of the home had been changed from convalescent to permanent, and he had been content with this. Six weeks later he had settled in well but some more homeopathic help was felt to be needed.

The difficulty at this point was that, in spite of eating regularly and adequately, he was still losing weight, and had developed a tendency towards looseness of the bowels, slipping occasionally into frank diarrhoea. There was complete control of the bowels at all times. No blood or mucus had been observed in the motion and the doctor ruled out the possibility of cancer on clinical grounds. Gaertner Bach 30c night and morning for three days was given. This produced a rapid benefit. The motions returned to normal within four days and after ten days no more weight had been lost. After a further ten days there had been a weight gain of 2.8kg. This remained the situation for about four months when the weight loss started again, although the bowels remained normal. Gaertner Bach 30c was given again, this time night and morning for three doses and the situation resolved, with the lost weight being regained. This became the pattern for the remaining two years of his life. Gaertner Bach 30c as above was required on three occasions and was successful each time. Death was due to cardiac failure.

Discussion

There is little doubt that Tuberculinum was the correct constitutional remedy for this patient. The low potency was selected because of his age and his perceived weakness at that time. Both the Arnica and the Opium were used as required for their specific indications in the acute situation. The major change and imbalance that was induced in the body's metabolism following the fall obviously manifested itself via the bowels and the weight loss, and the appropriate nosode was able to address this. Part of the picture of Gaertner Bach exactly matches the symptoms found here and this is an example of using a bowel nosode as a remedy in its own right. The fact that control rather than cure was all that was obtained was probably due to the age and inherent weakness of the patient. There are also the interesting connections of Tuberculinum being an associated remedy of Gaertner Bach, and the whole pattern of events having been initiated following weight loss, albeit not overtly pathological in origin.

CASE 9.3 Limping through life

The young dog's mobility is curtailed by chronic foot problems over several years. Conventional treatment provides only temporary relief and it is not until homeopathic treatment including a bowel nosode is employed that a permanent solution is found

A four year old entire male Labrador was obtained by his owners at six weeks old and received his first vaccination at eight weeks of age and his second at twelve weeks with both injections containing the full range of antigens. There were no apparent ill effects from these and routine worming was carried out as well using a prescription product. At five months old he developed a mildly irritant rash on his posterior abdomen. This was diagnosed as demodectic mange although no mites were found on skin scrapings. Treatment consisted of one injection of a long acting steroid (Depo-medrone, with a clinical action over three weeks) and application of an anti mange shampoo (Aludex) on three occasions at weekly intervals and the condition resolved. At one year old the dog developed a front leg lameness involving both legs with no clear indication of any laterality. A diagnosis of Osteocondritis Dissecans affecting the right shoulder joint and left elbow was made via x-ray and treatment with non steroidal anti-inflammatory drugs was instigated, several being tried with limited beneficial effect. At this stage the owner self prescribed a regime of Rhus Tox 6c once daily for the dog, which appeared to give some relief although the dog's exercise tolerance was reduced due to an ongoing degree of lameness. However, this was deemed to be a considerable improvement on the conventional drugs and hence the homeopathic remedy was continued on a regular basis. At around two years old the dog developed interdigital cysts on both front legs. The owner could not remember which foot was affected first but by the time homeopathic treatment was sought the outer digits of both legs were chronically affected with no significant difference in intensity between the two. One or other of the feet were flaring constantly resulting in the dog being acutely and virtually continuously lame. At no time were the hind legs affected. Treatment with antibiotics and steroids had been given on various occasions with only temporary relief of the most acute symptoms. The owner had ceased seeking such help and for the eight months prior to the consultation the only treatment had been by the bathing of the cysts in plain water as appropriate.

Physical examination posed no problems and revealed a patch of slightly moist eczema of approximately one inch diameter in the mid line near the base of the tail. Such discharge as there was appeared clear and the lesion was only mildly irritant. Anal glands were clear and although the dog had had much wax production from his ears all his life this had never caused him any problems. The only other skin involvement was a flat wart on the head adjacent to the left ear. All four feet were described as being 'constantly sweaty'. No other physical abnormalities were detected although the dog, in spite of being within the normal size for a Labrador, was considered to be very definitely at the lower end of the normal weight range. He was described as being a 'laid back, lazy dog, placid but timid', liking other dogs more than people. There was no overt fear of noise but he preferred a quiet life generally and would move away from too much hectic activity around him. Physical contact was sought and cuddles were enjoyed. In the consulting room he settled easily and went to sleep after the examination. He appeared to be keen to go for a walk in spite of being described as 'lazy' but the lameness made any assessment of that difficult. Heat was disliked and cool was sought actively. He enjoyed swimming and the owner felt that sea bathing gave a definite but temporary benefit. His appetite was very good (as with most Labradors!) but he would not eat raw meat or tomatoes. His normal diet was a tinned commercial food augmented by vegetables and other 'extras' as available. Eggs produced marked flatulence and carrots caused an aggravation of the feet. He loved milk and would not drink water unless it was flavoured with milk, when he would drink in large quantities. There was a marked desire for salty things.

Stopping the daily dose of Rhus Tox and an initial prescription of Silica 30c night and morning for three days produced no response of any kind. A re-examination of the case and a full repertorisation indicated Silica, Nat Mur, Calc Carb, Pulsatilla and Phosphorus as including the indicated remedy but it was considered that of those, Silica was still the remedy of choice. Accordingly, Gaertner Bach 30c night and morning for two days was prescribed, followed immediately by another three days of Silica 30c night and morning. After three weeks the owner reported that the cysts had started to dry up initially and to heal but had become moist again in the last week. However, the sore on the tail had healed and the dog was generally brighter and able to walk further. Silica 200c night and morning for three doses was given and the paws dried once more and proceeded to heal completely over the next two weeks. The lameness attributed to the osteocondritis decreased and after a month the dog was walking what were considered to be normal distances. There were no more cysts and a return of the general front leg lameness after three months was resolved with a further three doses of Silica 200c in twenty four hours. The wart remained and the ears continued to produce much wax but with no clinical problems.

Discussion

A theme of suppression runs through this case including the palliative use of a homeopathic remedy. The initial prescription of Silica was based partly on clinical experience of the condition, albeit as a local prescription, partly on the impression of the dog plus the likely aetiology of vaccination. As a result of the apparent failure of the remedy a repertorisation (Synthesis) was carried out using the rubrics:

MIND – Mildness
MIND – Affectionate
GENERALS – food and drink-salt-desires
GENERALS – food and drink-milk-desires
GENERALS – food and drink-meat-aversion
GENERALS – cold-ameliorates
GENERALS – heated becoming aggravates
EAR – wax-increased
EXTREMATIES – perspiration-foot
EXTREMATIES – swelling-foot

It could be argued that the mental symptoms are too similar and that the general symptoms selected rely too heavily on the food and drink section of the 'Generalities' chapter but these were among the most clear cut symptoms available. Also 'ailments from vaccination' could have been included. Be that as it may, the outcome, depending on the method of analysis employed (excluding small remedies and rubrics), produced the two remedies Nat Mur and Silica as alternating at the top of the analyses, with Calc Carb, Pulsatilla and Phosphorus also to be considered. Further consideration of the case confirmed the initial impression of Silica as the remedy of choice. The use of the associated bowel nosode was on the accepted indication of 'where a well indicated remedy fails to act or acts only for a short time', and Silica is a leading remedy of the Gaertner Bach group. The complete lack of response to the initial prescription was not felt to be due to too low a potency and hence merely moving up to a 200c did not appear to be indicated. The technique of following the nosode immediately with the remedy is based on the clinical experience that the closer the two remedies are given, the greater will be the synergistic effect. The unblocking of the remedy's action and the subsequent progress of the case confirmed the approach and comparison of the case with the remedy picture of Gaertner Bach shows that there was in fact a deep seated connection to the nosode.

It should be noted that Phosphorus is another leading remedy of the Gaertner Bach group and that Pulsatilla is listed as well, although Calc Carb and Nat Mur are not included. Perhaps a better repertorisation would have produced only associated remedies (although the Calcarea and Natrum salts are represented well in the group)!

10

BACILLUS NO. 7

Traditionally associated remedies
Arsenicum Iod, *Bromium*, Calc Iod, Ferrum Iod, **Iodum**, Kali Bich, Kali Brom, **Kali Carb**, Kali Nit, Merc Iod, Natrum Iod.

General considerations

The group was so named only because it was the seventh group of NLFB to be identified. Bacillus No. 10 was named for the same reason, but it must be remembered that there is in fact no connection between the groups other than an accidental similarity of nomenclature. The halogen elements iodine and bromine are found associated with the Bacillus No. 7 group.

Both iodine and bromine exist as remedies in their own right; Iodum is a leading remedy of the Bacillus No. 7 group, and Bromium is present in the second degree. Chlorine and fluorine are found in compounds which are used homeopathically, and are found associated with other bowel nosodes. All four of these halogens have themes connected with boundaries; chlorine at one end is often the victim of broken boundaries whilst at the other fluorine is more concerned with actually breaking boundaries and taboos (Scholten 1996). Iodine and bromine lie between these two extremes. This represents a syphilitic tendency that finds expression also in the presence of emaciation in the clinical pictures of the remedies containing a halogen. Additionally a tubercular connection is seen in many of the same remedies. There is an affinity with glands of various types. All the halogens are intrinsically hot elements in the homeopathic sense, with a sensitivity to, and aggravation from, exposure to external heat.

Iodum is certainly one of the hottest, if not the hottest, remedy in the materia medica, and its influence means that all remedies containing the element show the characteristic aggravation from heat. The general affinity for glands seen in the halogens finds its main expression in the case of iodine via a connection to the thyroid gland. Emaciation linked to great appetite is a feature of the remedy Iodum, and on the mental level there is often great concern that the patient will not be able to get enough to eat. The element often introduces a characteristic activity and restlessness into remedies. At the same time the opposite polarity of the element may be seen, producing lethargy and under- activity. Hence both hyper- and hypothyroidism may be influenced by the remedy.

In contrast, bromine is the most narcotic of the halogens. In many circumstances it is interchangeable with chlorine in the body, and the excretion of bromine is in inverse proportion to the chlorine intake (Carr 2007). Like the other members of the halogens it exerts a tubercular influence, but displays more of a sycotic emphasis than the others in the group. It is associated with both lymph and endocrine glands, exhibiting hardness of affected structures. There is a major involvement in conditions affecting the endocrine system, with the endocrine gland most affected being the anterior lobe of the pituitary. Another area where its effects are seen is the respiratory system.

Both of these elements are found as major constituents of the associated remedies of Bacillus No. 7, yet some of their major features, such as the hyperactivity of iodine, are absent from the clinical picture of the nosode. This led John Paterson (1936) to consider that the major influence within the remedy group came from the potassium that is also well represented. This view is supported by the presence of Kali Carb. in the associated group. There is a strong connection of the carbonates with the Morgan Pure group of remedies and Kali Carb. is indeed represented in that group, but only in the first degree. However, it is the combination with potassium that overrides the carbonate influence and places the remedy firmly in the Bacillus No. 7 group as a leading remedy.

John Paterson's survey revealed 0.82% of NLFB connected to Bacillus No 7. Elizabeth Paterson reported 2.72% for it in the clinical situation. Bacillus No 7. was found in 1.15% of samples from the dogs but the group was not found in cats. The timescale of the samples as discussed in Chapter 7, together with their size, should both be considered in the interpretation of these results, but it is clear that the incidence of clinical indications for the nosode is similar to many of the other groups.

The themes of Bacillus No 7. are 'mental and physical fatigue' together with 'stiffness and rigidity'. Clarke (1982) states that 'The Potassium salts have more specific relation to the solid tissues than the fluids of the body: to the blood corpuscles rather than to the blood plasma. The fibrous tissues are particularly affected . . .'. The weakness associated with the Kali salts generally is reflected in the nosode and the neuromuscular junction is a major site of its action. Potassium also has a direct action on the heart. In addition to the remedies listed in Chapter 2, Calcarea Hypophosphorosa has been associated with the nosode (Blasig and Vint 2001) and the general lack of tone in the musculoskeletal system leads, certainly in animals, to a look very like the sagging appearance associated with a need for Causticum (which is itself a potassium salt). In miasmatic terms the strongest link is with psora, although features of the other two basic miasms are also present.

Materia medica

The general pattern is one of fatigue and lethargy with the principle modalities of being worse for standing, movement, draughts, cold and damp. There is amelioration from rest and warmth.

Mentally there is great disinclination to make any effort at all, accompanied by tiredness and tension. In spite of this, megalomania is occasionally seen, but in the main the mere thought of having to make any effort, mental or physical, is enough to bring on feelings of weakness. The onset of symptoms is usually gradual and patients can appear prematurely aged. This lack of activity runs through the function of the whole body and is at the root of most of the symptoms. Sleep is light, restless and unrefreshing, showing the typical Kali characteristic of difficulty getting to sleep and waking in the early hours of the morning.

Headaches are of the dull variety and there is catarrhal deafness.

The digestive system exhibits this lack of functional tone with generally weak digestive processes, resulting in a sense of fullness after food and flatulence in both the stomach and abdomen. There is much eructation from the stomach but little passage of wind from the rectum. Vomiting is rarely seen. There is pain in the region of the liver due to the poor digestion. There is an aversion to fats because of the digestive problems associated with them. The normal state is one of constipation.

The cardiovascular system is characterised by a slow pulse and a tendency to hypotension. Weakness of heart muscle can lead to sudden cardiac arrest. Faintness and vertigo occur following standing for too long or exertion. Sudden exertion produces syncope. The lack of tone in the circulation leads to puffiness and some oedema in the skin, particularly of the face and eyelids. There is a tendency to chilliness with sensitivity to cold and damp but at the other extreme there may be excessive perspiration. Weakness in the blood vessels results in bursting of veins, especially in the fingers, and haemorrhoids. There is a tendency to thrombosis of the central retinal vein.

The respiratory system is affected by asthma and there is bronchitis with thick mucus and difficult expectoration that is worse at 2.00a.m. The bronchitis is accompanied by chest pains. Quinsy and tonsillitis with swelling of the throat is seen.

Loss of function characterises the genital system in both sexes, and in the female there is pain in the vulva. At the same time all genital discharges may be profuse. Uterine bleeding may also be present. Urine flow is weak.

Poor muscle tone generally gives weakness and stiffness and there may be atrophy of particular muscle groups. Movement is thus slow and laboured. Wrists and ankles become fixed and all joints can show swelling and pain. Osteo-, rheumatoid and periarthritis are found, potentially involving any area of the body. The neck and shoulder regions are particularly affected in humans, with a characteristic 'cracking' of the affected joints, but in animals osteoarthritis in the stifle (knee) is seen specifically. Faintness from standing for too long can occur due to pain in the back. Shooting pains in the legs, fixation of the left hip and night-time cramps occur. Pain in the feet may be associated with gout in either big toe, although it is more common in the left. Patients often appear as flatfooted. Abdominal prolapse due to muscle weakness can occur.

Oedematous plaques may occur in the skin and cracks in the skin of the hands and heat in the palms are seen. Ganglia and nodules occur on the hands.

BACILLUS No. 7	
Mind	Mental lethargy. Tiredness. Tension.
Head	Dull headaches.
Face	Catarrhal deafness. Prematurely aged look.
Abdomen	Lack of muscle tone. Constipation. Feeling bloated after eating. Flatulence relieved by belching. Pain near liver. Prolapses.
Appetite	Aversion to and < fats.
Cardiovascular	Slow heart beat. Hypotension. Weakness of heart muscle. Exertion produces syncope, faintness and vertigo. Bursting of veins. Haemorrhoids. Thrombosis of central retinal vein.
Urogenital	Loss of sexual function. Pain in vulva. Profuse genital discharges. Uterine bleeding. Weak urine flow.
Respiratory	Asthma. Bronchitis with thick mucus and difficult expectoration. Chest pains. Tonsillitis with swelling of throat.

BACILLUS No. 7 (continued)	
Musculoskeletal	Poor muscle tone. Weakness and stiffness. Slow movement. Atrophy of muscle groups. Swollen, painful, fixed joints. 'Cracking' of neck and shoulder joints. Pain in back from standing. Cramps at night.
Sleep	Light, restless, unrefreshing. Difficulty getting to sleep. Wakes early.
Skin	Cracks on hands. Ganglia and nodules on hands.
Modalities & Generalities	< Standing, movement, draughts, cold and damp. 2.00a.m. > Rest, warmth. Both hypo- and hyperthyroidism may be helped.

CASE 10.1   A difficult patient

An injury tips a horse into an acute pathological expression of its constitutional type. The appropriate remedy gives considerable success but it is not until the prescription of the associated bowel nosode that the full benefits are seen.

Homeopathic treatment was sought for a seven-year-old neutered hunter type male horse who had developed a generalised sensitivity to touch and suspicion of humans following a soft tissue injury. He was a big-boned horse, 16.1 hands (1.65m) tall to the top of his shoulders. He had come to his present home three years previously with a view to being used for recreational riding plus some low level competition work. He was stabled on a yard of around twenty other horses, towards whom he appeared largely indifferent. He had settled well when he arrived but had subsequently proved somewhat of a disappointment. He had never worked well and was difficult to handle, in spite of the owner being an experienced rider. He would sweat easily all over after little movement and although essentially friendly, he would occasionally bite and kick out at both people and other horses, especially when the saddle and bridle were being put on, even resenting a head collar. He was described as having 'poor conformation' and although his back had been examined on several occasions by both a veterinary surgeon and a chiropractor, nothing significant had been found to be amiss. He was sensitive to being groomed, being very restless throughout the procedure. He was apprehensive when being shod, although not appearing dangerous. The appetite was good and there had been no major health problems over the time that he had been with the present owners. Equally, no health problems had been reported by the vendors. He had been vaccinated and wormed regularly, and although he disliked being injected was manageable on those occasions.

About one month prior to the consultation the horse had been involved in a fight with another horse and had, as a result of a kick, sustained a flesh wound to the mid thigh on the lateral aspect of the left hind leg. It had been treated conventionally with antibiotics and had healed normally, if rather slowly. The owners had been instructed to bathe it, and this they had found extremely difficult due to the great sensitivity that had developed around the wound, even when it was healing well. There had been a corresponding increase in sensitivity over the whole body. At the time of the homeopathic consultation it was impossible to touch the left thigh anywhere. All attempts to saddle up were met with more resistance than ever before, and the owner had given up all attempts to ride him.

At the time of the consultation it was impossible to carry out a detailed physical examination in safety, any contact resulting in a violent reaction from the horse. He was, however, happy to have people around provided there was no attempt to touch him. Visual examination confirmed of the wound revealed that it had healed well with no excessive flesh. Eating and drinking were normal, as were urination and defaecation. He was wary of other horses coming too near.

He was unwilling to let anyone look him straight in the eye. If it was attempted whilst he was in his box he would immediately turn through one hundred and eighty degrees and stand facing the wall. There was no tendency to kick at these times, just a firm refusal to return anyone's gaze. With hindsight the owner said that he had always had a reluctance about eye contact but that it had never been as bad as it was at that time.

The general impression was that his general movement was ungainly and un-coordinated, but that there was no hint of any definite lameness, certainly not involving the injured leg.

Arnica 1M was given initially, one dose night and morning for three doses, on the basis of the condition having been triggered by an injury plus the sensitivity to touch. This produced no effect and after two weeks the prescription was changed to Kali Carb. 30c, night and morning for three days. This was selected taking into account the extreme sensitivity to touch, the behaviour pattern of turning on people with whom he was basically friendly, and the ease with which the horse began to sweat.

After a further three weeks there had been some definite improvement. He was still sensitive generally, resenting being touched, but the area around where the wound had been was no longer more sensitive than elsewhere. He would still avoid eye contact. He was reported as being brighter in himself. Such improvement as there had been had occurred in the first week after the remedy, and was being maintained.

The remedy was repeated at 200c, three doses in twenty-four hours and this restarted and accelerated the improvement. After two weeks there was still some sensitivity to touch but it had reduced by about fifty percent. He appeared to be more friendly generally and although still not keen on eye contact, would now only turn his head away rather than his whole body. He now accepted a head collar without protest, but there had been no attempt to put a saddle on. As before, the improvement had been rapid after the administration of the remedy and had now ceased. The Kali Carb. was repeated as above and after a further three weeks all excessive sensitivity had gone, saddling and riding were managed without problems and there was no longer any reluctance to eye contact. No further treatment was given at this stage.

Some two and a half months later the problems with eye contact were returning, with a little bit of bad behaviour beginning again whilst being ridden. Kali Carb. at a1M potency was administered as three doses in twenty-four hours. Although there was no further deterioration, there was not the improvement that had been expected. After a month Bacillus No. 7 200c was prescribed night and morning for three days. All the returning symptoms were resolved within ten days and did not return. In addition there was a marked improvement in the horse generally, described by the owner as 'he has never looked so good or moved so well'.

Discussion

This horse was obviously in a basically Kali Carb. state at the time of receiving the injury, and that challenge tipped the balance into an acute form of the underlying constitutional condition. The successive doses of the remedy initially produced the desired effect but the failure of the 1M potency, in spite of having some effect, to take the case forward indicated a reassessment of the situation. An increase to 10M would have been one option, or perhaps the introduction of a potency chord from 200c through 1M to 10M, thereby allowing the horse to select the exact potency it required at a particular time. The author's view is that this is how potency chords probably work, with the exact resonance being selected by the patient from those available within the chord. The idea that a potency chord allows a low potency to address the physical aspects of a case, the intermediate ones to affect the functional aspects while the higher ones work at the mental level (Pedalino 2006), does not entirely fit in this case, as the higher potencies had already been employed with limited success. In practice the author's liking for bowel nosodes led him immediately in their direction. It should be noted that it was after the use of the bowel nosode that the owner reported the final improvement in the horse's condition, compatible with a general 'tightening up' of the ligaments and tendons of the body.

An interesting aspect of this symptom picture was the unwillingness to make eye contact, expressed in the extreme form of turning completely away. That this was part of the disease picture is beyond doubt, but there is no mention of it in the materia medicas under Kali Carb. However, in the Mind chapter of the repertory (Synthesis) is a rubric 'Delusion – faces sees – ugly (hideous)', in which Kali Carb. is listed in the second degree. Considerations of delusions do not normally form part of the veterinary approach to remedy selection, and did not in this case, but perhaps it is an aspect that should not be so lightly dismissed, even though its applications are obviously limited.

CASE 10.2   Exhausted after being 'cured'

After a long history of ill health, a lady is promised that a hysterectomy will resolve her problems. Post operatively she experiences continued problems until a bowel nosode provides the answer.

A fifty-four-year-old married lady had two sons, the elder aged thirty-four and the younger twenty-seven. She had married at the age of nineteen and her first child was born fifteen months later. The couple had planned for other children, but a seven-year gap was more than had been intended and no more pregnancies occurred after the second one, in spite of all efforts. No chemical contraception had ever been used. About five years after the birth of the second child, the lady began to experience gynaecological problems which increased as she became older. Various investigations of and treatments for her problems had taken place over the years, but the exact details, and the diagnoses, were not remembered clearly. Sometimes there had been some temporary relief, and whilst the possibility of a hyster-ectomy had been mentioned on several occasions, that option had been declined each time. In addition to the reproductive symptoms, occasional acute attacks of cystitis had occurred and these had been treated with antibiotics as necessary. A degree of urinary incontinence had also appeared as time progressed, and hot flushes and bouts of depression accompanied by outbursts of anger had developed in recent years. About a year prior to the homeopathic consultation, the whole situation had worsened, with abdominal pain becoming a feature. A hysterectomy had been carried out some three months later following a diagnosis of uterine fibroids. Since that time, she had experienced continuous marked lassitude and exhaustion, the urinary incontinence had worsened and there had been further attacks of cystitis. Antibiotics had been prescribed as appropriate. The bouts of depression had persisted, with a steady worsening of her temper, which could now flare at any time. Although a wide range of vitamin supplements had been self prescribed and taken over the ten months since the operation, there had been no improvement in the mental state. Apart from antibiotics, all other offers of medication had been declined, and it was when anti depressant drugs were suggested that, through desperation rather than conviction, homeopathic help had been sought.

The lady was small and petite, and even by such standards had always been considered to be thin. Her appetite was described as 'normal' and she had never shown any tendency to put any on any weight. At one stage in the past her thyroid function had been inves-tigated via blood sample (??T4 estimation only), and pronounced to be within normal limits. This test had been repeated since the oper-ation and the thyroid had been considered still to be functioning normally. Her thirst was small. Until recently she had always been lively and optimist, enjoying holidays and an active social life at home. However, at the time of the consultation, even when not actively depressed she had no great enthusiasm for life. She confessed that, although loving her family, when depressed she now regretted giving up her intention to train as a nurse in order to get married. Her elder son had never been a problem beyond the expected upsets of adolescence, and was now married with two children and in steady employment. Her grandchildren were giving her increasing pleasure as they got older, although she had not been keen on them when they were very young. Her younger son, however, had always been somewhat of a worry, both physically and mentally. He had a somewhat chequered medical history in childhood, the main features being appendicitis, osteomyelitis and eczema. Even as an adult his eczema would flare up periodically and he seemed incapable of settling into a stable adult life, drifting from job to job with periods of unemployment. His personal life was no more stable. The aspect that upset his mother most was that he seemed to have no concerns about his lifestyle, and saw no need to change. He still lived at home. Medical opinion was that the depression was largely due to stress based on her anxiety over her son.

Other than for her son, she had no significant worries or fears. Generally, she slept well although she felt tired in spite of that. She rarely dreamt, but sometimes woke early and could not sleep again for thinking about herself and the family, although not exclusively about their health. There had been no significant change in her weight since the operation. Apart from the gynaecological problems, there were no significant events in her medical history. She was an only child and both her parents had enjoyed good health and died of natural causes in old age. The medical history of her more extended family was similarly unremarkable.

She used to be an organised, tidy person, but this had been largely overridden by her condition, which had produced a 'can't be bothered' attitude. Occasionally she would do some tidying, but soon stopped because it made her even more tired than usual.

She had a great liking for heat and in the summer she would lie for hours in the sun, without becoming either excessively tanned or burnt. Wind in all forms, even slight draughts and warm summer breezes, were disliked. Her appetite and thirst were unaffected. She had no marked food aversions and was happy to eat most things. There was a strong desire for butter and salt. Flatulence was not a problem and motions were normal. Physically the wound had healed well and there was no longer any abdominal pain. In addition to the lassitude, the physical problems of the incontinence and the cystitis remained.

Sepia 30c was prescribed night and morning for four days. This was selected partly on the basis of 'never well since a hysterectomy'. (In the veterinary world this is a recognised aetiology following neutering of mature females. In animals it is always a panhysterectomy that is performed, with the ovaries being removed, but it was felt that the similarity of aetiology justified the choice in spite of any slight differences there may have been in the procedure.) Features such as the regrets over her lost training, the depression and anger, the liking for heat and the incontinence also indicated the remedy.

Two days after finishing the Sepia she experienced an attack of cystitis for which, unfortunately, she resorted once more to antibiotics. This settled quickly, but after three weeks there had been no improvement in her overall condition, thereby reducing further what hope she had for help from homeopathy. With difficulty she was persuaded to try the Sepia 30c once more, and accordingly a course of three doses over twenty four hours was given, with her promising not to rush to antibiotics if the cystitis recurred. In the event there was no such reaction and after a month she reported that the incontinence was less, there had been no cystitis, and her mood had somewhat improved – this latter being confirmed emphatically by her husband!

Her scepticism about homeopathy had now been replaced by something approaching a 'one more tablet will do it' attitude, more in keeping with her old temperament. This was, however, considered to be too optimistic, as the lassitude and easy exhaustion were unchanged. Therefore, a further course of three doses of Sepia 30c over twenty-four hours was administered. This produced no additional beneficial effect, although the previous improvement was maintained. After another month the potency of the Sepia was increased to 200c and three doses over twenty-four hours were given as before. The main effect was a further positive change in attitude, but the persisting weakness precluded a full return to her old self. The incontinence may or may not have improved, but her new found optimism made accurate assessment difficult.

At this point the remedy was changed to Bacillus No. 7, 30c night and morning for three days. The prescription was based on the theme of mental and physical fatigue found with the nosode. Over the next six weeks there was a steady improvement in her energy levels, at the end of which time she considered herself to be back to normal. This has been maintained, there has been no more cystitis and all that remains is a slight degree of 'acceptable' incontinence.

Discussion

Sepia fitted the pattern of this case miasmatically, with the marked focus of the historical symptoms on the reproductive system indicating a predominant sycosis. Other additional features of the presenting totality suggested that the lady was in a Sepia state. Its successful use confirmed the choice, but as the case progressed it appeared not to be the complete answer. The Bacillus No. 7 was prescribed as a remedy in its own right to address the then predominantly psoric element in the case. It is, however, likely that it acted in part as a direct augmentation of the action of the Sepia, as it is now established that Sepia should be included as an associated remedy of Bacillus No. 7 (see Appendix).

CASE 10.3   Overcoming a bad start

A puppy develops a developmental problem following vaccination. The use of a vaccination nosode and other remedies restores much of the situation but a bowel nosode is required before matters are completely resolved.

A seven-month-old female Newfoundland puppy was presented for homeopathic treatment with a severe failure to develop normally. The puppy had been obtained from a reputable breeder at eight weeks of age, having been selected from, the litter because of her large size which was what was wanted. Initially all was well, she was lovely and friendly, eating well and growing normally. She received her first routine vaccination (distremper, adenovirus, parvovirus and lepto-spirosis) at ten weeks old and the second two weeks later with no apparent ill effects.

From around four months of age she had become progressively slower and her appetite decline significantly. She ceased to play voluntarily and refused to walk. Drinking was described as normal and there was no bowel upset. There had been no sign of the first season. She would seek heat, continued to be friendly and enjoyed fuss. Although her skeleton had continued to grow the rate had slowed and become uneven with the hind legs growing more than the front. The hind legs were 'cow hocked' with both hocks turned inwards. Both front legs showed extreme dropping of the carpi to the extent that the posterior surface of each was in contact with the ground. And both legs were turning outwards from the knees (wrists). There was no excessive thickening of the lower ends of the radii and no pain on palpation. Muscular development over the whole body was poor. The oral mucosa was a good colour and refill time was good. The coat was thin but there was no pruritis

A conventional diagnosis of 'nutritional deficiency and imbalance caused by an unknown metabolic disorder' had led to oral mineral and vitamin supplementation with injections of anabolic steroid (Nandoral). This produced no benefit and the case had been referred to an orthopaedic specialist who considered there was 'irreversible tendon and ligament weakness with possible growth plate insufficiency'. X-ray had revealed the cortex of the bones to have been 'slightly thinner than he would have wished'. His advice was surgery to fix and immobilise the joints of the front legs with steel pins, advice which was rejected and homeopathic treatment sought.

A blood showed normal liver and kidney function ad all parameters within normal limits. A second sample was submitted for specialist thyroid investigation in the USA. Treatment was begun with Canine Combination Nosode (source material the conventional multi-vaccine in standard use) 30c b d for five days, to be followed by Calc Flour 30c b d for one week. At re-examination after three weeks later the dog was eating well again but still quiet. The hocks were possibly a little straighter (wishful thinking?) but there was certainly no change in the front legs. Such improvement as there had been had begun within three days of commencing the nosode but had now ceased. Calc Flour 30c was continued at the rate of one dose on alternate days for a further two weeks. One week later the results of the American sample gave a diagnosis of 'acute thyroiditis, probably due to vaccination'.

One month later the appetite had returned to normal, the hocks now showed definite improvement and the front legs had also improved but were not yet right. The puppy, however, was still quiet and easily tired if encouraged to play/walk and progress now was extremely slow compared to previously. Bacillus no. 7 30c b d for three days was prescribed to be followed by Calc Flour 30c o d for one week then Ruta 30c o d for ten days. Three weeks later there was a normally lively puppy and all legs continued to improve. No further treatment was given. Six weeks later all appeared to be normal and the first season occurred at eleven months of age

Discussion

The tentative diagnosis based on 'Never Well Since' was confirmed by both the blood test and the response to treatment with the nosode. Calc Flour was selected on its general properties including the initial discrepancy between the front and hind legs. Although successful as far as the developmental aspects were concerned, the systemic effect of the tiredness and weakness was unaffected, hence the introduction of the bowel nosode with its keynote of weakness and easy exhaustion rather than an increase in the potency of the Calc Flour. The remedy is also included in the amended associated remedies list so an additional benefit may have been obtained from that. The Ruta was added for further support in view of its particular affinity for joints and the soft tissues surrounding them.

11

BACILLUS NO. 10

Traditionally associated remedy
Calc Fluor.

General considerations

Although regarded generally as one of the more minor of the bowel nosodes, Bacillus No 10, in the author's opinion, deserves a greater prominence than it has been given hitherto. There are certain aspects of its remedy picture that have particular relevance to some of the human conditions found in modern western societies as well as broader indications across all species.

John Paterson did not identify any of the bacteria related to the nosode in his survey, but Elizabeth Paterson encountered it in 1.52% of her clinical cases: it did not feature at all in the similar but more restricted animal survey (see Chapter 2). Other workers have reported similar low occurrences. Add to this the fact that Calc. Fluor. has been the only remedy associated traditionally with it and its reputation as a minor bowel nosode is not surprising.

Fluorine, the most reactive and syphilitic of the halogens, is undoubtedly a major influence in the nosode. The reactivity of the element means that it is not found in its free state in nature, but only in combination. It gives great hardness to compounds that contain it and conditions that require remedies containing it exhibit the same hardness in the patient's tissues. The syphilitic influence shows on the mental level as a letting go of values and the breaking of boundaries, whilst physically this manifests as a loss of form and structure. Fluorine is involved particularly with bones, joints and teeth.

This has led to the interpretation that there is a predominantly syphilitic bias to Bacillus No 10: Calc. Fluor. is listed by Banerjea (2003) as an antisyphilitic remedy in the second degree. However, the Calc. Fluor. remedy picture, in addition to its syphilitic aspects, shows some significant sycotic features such as the tendency towards exostosis formation and glandular enlargements accompanied by hardness of the tissue. In his original work John Paterson found that the two remedies most closely connected to the appearance of the appropriate NLFB were Thuja and Nat Sulph., both of which remedies have strong links to the sycotic miasm and are listed by Banerjea as anti-sycotic remedies in the third degree. In addition, Thuja has some lesser but definite syphilitic aspects, particularly in the mental sphere (dreams of death, dying etc).

Therefore Bacillus No. 10 has a much stronger sycotic influence than is indicated by considering Calc. Fluor. as its only associated remedy and should be regarded as having a sycotic/syphilitic/psoric balance. It is quoted in connection with the treatment of ringworm, a predominantly sycotic condition and one for which Nat. Sulph. is a frequently prescribed and successful remedy in practice. Other remedies mentioned by John Paterson as having a possible association with the nosode are Aralia Rac., Calc. Phos., Kali Bic. and Sepia (Agrawal 1995), and all of these exhibit a sycotic/syphilis balance in varying degrees. Similar consideration of the expanded associated remedy list (see Appendix) indicates a continuation of this trend.

In general miasmatic terms the combination of the predominant sycotic and syphilitic influences represents the situation encountered in clinical cases of cancer (Saxton 2006), with the proliferation of new abnormal tissue linked to the destruction of both existing physical boundaries and normal tissue. Thus, although the exact miasmatic balance will vary with the individual case, Bacillus No 10 may have a role as part of the management regime in some cases of neoplasia, with its possible use being as an intercurrent remedy.

Modern clinical experience suggests that Platina should be added to the list of remedies associated with Bacillus No 10. In this context it may be relevant to reflect on the issues around size that are found in the Platina picture, especially the sensation/delusion concerned with 'largeness', and there are also connections to extremes of appetite including 'bulimia caused by boredom' and guilt feelings at having eaten to much. Other recent clinical experience indicates that Sabal also deserves inclusion as an associated remedy.

Materia medica

A major sycotic influence is seen in many cases as a generally hurried and excessive approach to life and a need to be always 'on the go'. Mentally this is not always the restlessness of real or imagined anxiety but rather a more positive need, bordering on compulsion, to find yet another task to do. However, there may be also the characteristic of an overactive mind linked with anxiety and sadness to the extent of depression, which may show either as general irritability or as a particular hypersensitivity to criticism. A trait of compulsive obsessive behaviour runs through the type which can take different forms, ranging from a rigid insistence on fixed routines over trifles to more extreme manifestations. Commonly seen forms are an over strict concentration on cleanliness or an absolute devotion to exercise in any form, be it the gymnasium, running or any other activity-in extreme cases the whole of the patient's life may revolve around this routine and there is often a strong competitive urge in any sporting activities undertaken.

Anxiety, obsession, depression and sensitivity to criticism may come together in an undue concern about body shape and size, leading in extreme cases to a situation where nothing in the way of exercise or even cosmetic surgery is ever enough. This can be exacerbated further by a tendency in the nosode's type to non specific eating disorders. There can be an inexplicable loss of appetite or marked lack of interest in food and this may become linked to more delusionary aspects as indicated above to produce clinical conditions such as anorexia whilst at the other extreme bulimia may be seen occasionally. It has been suggested (Malcolm 2007) that this may originate in fears about ageing and/or loss of sexual attraction and function.

Other symptoms include frontal headaches with congestive pain over the eyes, especially the left eye. The mouth produces halitosis and there is inflammation and sponginess of the gums associated with bleeding giving blood stained saliva. In humans the face may appear either ruddy or pale but this feature is not observable in animals.

Even when there is a normal appetite and overall adequate intake of food, a specific aversion to breakfast is found with attendant discomfort in the abdomen. Usually marked greed or gluttony is not seen at any time unless part of the syndrome of an eating disorder. Animals may be reluctant or refuse to eat at any time during the morning but show no such inhibitions later in the day. Dietary desires are strong for fried fish, sweets and chocolate, with aversions to eggs, bread, tomatoes and tea. Eggs and fats produce digestive upsets, principally nausea and vomiting, but in addition fats are likely to produce pain in the region of the gall bladder. Nausea and vomiting are seen but flatulence is not a feature. Motions are passed mainly early in the morning; they tend to be loose and in spite of a degree of urgency they are passed slowly. Inactivity of the rectum can produce constipation. There is irritation around the anus and tenderness around the coccyx, with animals showing persistent rubbing around the base of the tail and tenderness on palpation of the area. There are usually no lesions to account for the symptom but occasionally dermatitis may be present in the perianal region. Generally, in carnivores the anal glands are not affected.

The respiratory system is affected with thick mucous secretions, resulting in catarrh and cough with difficult expectoration. The cough is worse in the morning. Asthma occurs and patients may exhibit an adverse reaction to conventional medication given for the condition.

The sycotic influence is seen strongly in the genital system with leucorrhoea producing green, corrosive discharges with the fishy odour typical of sycosis. This is accompanied by irritation and swelling of the vulva with rawness and cracking of the skin in the groins. Cracking and irritation of the scrotum is found in the male along with involvement of the inguinal region. Increased sexual desire is seen. There is thickening of the urethra and frequent urination occurs without cystitis.

Rheumatism is seen most commonly in both thighs. Arthritis, when it occurs, affects especially the left knee (stifle in animals). There is pain in both iliac fossae.

The skin exhibits flat or pointed warts, which are found mainly on the hands and feet. Fatty cysts are seen on the neck and lipomas occur in the region of the lower ribs (rear ribs in animals), with panniculitis in the chest wall, although there is no significant laterality. Circinate eruptions on the

---

BACILLUS NO. 10

Mind	Overactive mind. Anxiety and depression. Irritability and sensitivity. Excessive and obsessional behaviours (cleanliness and exercise).
Head	Frontal headaches. Pain above eyes, especially left.
Face	Halitosis. Spongy gums. Bleeding gums. Bloody saliva.
Appetite	Loss of appetite. Aversion to breakfast. General eating disorders. Desire for fried fish, sweets and chocolate. Aversion to eggs, bread, tomatoes and tea.
Alimentary	Nausea, vomiting. Pain in gall bladder from fats. Loose motions. Motions passed early in morning. Urgency but stool passed slowly. Irritation around anus.
Urogenital	Leucorrhoea. Green corrosive discharges with fishy smell. Swelling and irritation of genitalia in both sexes. High libido. Frequent micturition without cystitis. Thickening of the urethra.

BACILLUS NO. 10 (continued)	
Respiratory	Cough < morning. Nasal catarrh. Thick mucus secretions with difficult expectoration. Asthma with adverse reactions to prescribed conventional medications.
Musculoskeletal	Rheumatism in thighs. Arthritis in left knee (stifle). Pain in iliac fossae.
Skin	Warts flat or pointed on hands and feet. Fatty cysts and lipomas. Ringworm. Circinate eruptions. Dermatitis of limbs and in flexures of joints. Pruritis without lesions, cracking and dermatitis in the inguinal region. Profuse perspiration from axillae.

hands, paronychia and dermatitis on the limbs, in the flexures of joints and around the inguinal region are found. Irritation of the inguinal region without obvious lesions is seen also. Excessive perspiration from the axillae is seen in humans and horses.

CASE 11.1 Life in the old dog yet

An active ex agility dog develops conditions common to the older animal. Conventional medication fails to relieve the situation. Initial homeopathic treatment results in some alleviation but it requires the use of a bowel nosode to achieve a significant improvement.

A fourteen year old entire male Border Collie was presented with a conventional diagnosis of severe prostatic hyperplasia and an adenoma (clinical assessment) some half inch in diameter located to the left of the anus. There had been some slight but noticeable weight loss over the previous six months; the owners had not been unduly worried about this as the dog had continued to eat and drink normally and they had regarded it as nothing more than a consequence of age. Passage of both faeces and urine was slow and accompanied by straining. The symptoms had been worsening over the previous three months. The faeces appeared normal and the urine was normal as determined by testing with a 'dipstick'. Rectal examination revealed an enlarged, hard but smooth prostate that was not painful on palpation. The adenoma was also painless on palpation. Clinical examination revealed no other abnormality.

Conventional treatment for both presenting symptoms had been by injections of delmadinone acetate (available as Tardak) at intervals of three weeks. This had been administered over the previous two months (three injections) with no observable improvement, and hence homeopathic help had been sought.

In earlier years there had been major involved in agility competitions, and the dog (and his owner) had enjoyed considerable success as he was both a talented and enthusiastic performer. Eight years prior to the present troubles he had been treated by the complementary practice for musculoskeletal problems which were interfering with his competitive performance. Conventional diagnosis via x-ray at that time had been one of spondylitis of the lumbar- sacral region with additional involvement of the left hip. Conventionally he had been prescribed a non steroidal anti inflammatory preparation containing meloxicam (Metacam) without long term benefit. A course of acupuncture and homeopathic treatment had resulted, over a six week period, in overcoming the need for the NSAID. Following this he had been retired from competition and had required only the occasional dose of Rhus Tox, by owner's self prescription, in subsequent years. One problem had been that the owners had other dogs involved in the agility circuit who required training and it had been difficult, if not impossible, to curb the dog's enthusiasm to be involved in that training.

He was described as a 'lively dog who loved life'. He got on well with the other two Border Collies in the house and there was no clear dominance in their relationship. He had no marked fears. His appetite was described as good rather than greedy and he would make no attempt to eat the other dogs' food once he had finished his own. His thirst was considered 'normal', although all three dogs shared a common water source. Feeding was with a commercial tinned food and no dietary desires or aversions could be identified. All the dogs were fed one meal daily in the evening, and were not offered food at any other time. The dogs were kept in the house as pets rather than in kennels but the owners could not specify any particular traits with regard to heat. In earlier years regular full vaccinations and wormings had been administered. All three dogs continued to be wormed regularly but the dog's vaccinations were limited now to Leptospirosis only on a more intermittent basis.

Initial treatment was with Thuja 30c, one night and morning for 4 days. This resulted in a general mental brightening, the owners having accounted for any previous slight quietness as a result of age. Urine flow became normal over the next month although passage of faeces continued to show some difficulty. The referring veterinary surgeon reported no marked change in the size of the prostate gland after further rectal examination and the adenoma was unchanged. There appeared to be some weight gain on subjective assessment but this was not marked. After a further two weeks the urinary symptoms reappeared and the surface of the adenoma appeared to be sore, although his brighter demeanour was maintained. At this stage the Tardak injections were being continued but the owners reported that the adenoma appeared to increase in size after each injection. Accordingly, after consultation with the referring veterinary surgeon, those injections were discontinued. The prescription was changed to Sabal 6c one daily for two weeks. Initially this eased the urinary symptoms once more but after one month this regressed to the original situation.

At this stage Bacillus No. 10, 30c night and morning for three days was prescribed. Within a week the urinary symptoms had improved slightly but the adenoma developed an increased level of superficial soreness, and became irritant: periodically the dog would lick fiercely at the anal area but would stop if told to do so. Sabal 6c was repeated with one dose daily for one week. The urinary symptoms had subsided completely ten days after finishing the course. The adenoma remained sore and developed two small areas which bled periodically, but apart from that he continued to be bright and happy in himself. Nitric Acid 30c night and morning for three days was prescribed followed by Thuja 30c once more, one night and morning for 4 days. The ulcers healed and the adenoma lost its soreness and began reducing, stabilizing at around half its original size after five weeks. A further two day course of Thuja 30c at that time produced no further effect. Rectal examination showed a reduction in the prostate of approximately one third and some softening on palpation. Both faeces and urine were being passed normally. The owner was happy to monitor the situation from this point with no further treatment. There was a slight return of the urinary symptoms after four months which were checked by five once daily doses of Sabal 6c. The adenoma remained small and non irritant. There was no further return of the symptoms for the remaining eleven months of the dog's life. Death was ascribed to 'natural causes' although no post mortem examinations were carried out.

Discussion

The initial prescription of Thuja was made on the general miasmatic considerations of benign hyperplasia, plus the slight indication of a possible left sided laterality based on the position of the adenoma. The anatomy of carnivores is such that the effect of pressure from an enlarged prostate is often as great on the rectum as on the urethra and hence the easing of the urine flow without a corresponding benefit to the passage of faeces is not surprising. The early improved mental picture would indicate that Thuja was a correct prescription. In view of the miasmatic basis for the initial prescription, Sycotic Co. could have been considered to be the more logical prescription of a bowel nosode, and it is, of course, unknown what the effect of such a prescription would have been. Bacillus No. 10 was preferred in part due to the dog's history of, and obvious liking for, physical activity, although it is arguable that such traits are found often in Border Collies. Other factors influencing the choice were the hardness of the prostate gland and the initial success of the Sabal, linked to the author's growing conviction of the associated relationship between that remedy and Bacillus No. 10. Nitric Acid, which resolved the bleeding from the adenoma, is also in the expanded associated remedy list for Bacillus No. 10. The soreness of the adenoma that developed could have been part of the aggravating effect of the final Tardak injection but the timing of its appearance is more likely to point to a more active effect from the use of the bowel nosode. The use of moderate and low potencies was decided on in view of the age of the dog (in spite of his apparent general fitness) and the pathological aspects of the condition. The final decision of the owner to 'let sleeping dogs lie' is not uncommon in veterinary practice and so what, if anything, could have been achieved with further treatment will never be known. However, the dog's subsequent health history would indicate that there had been a fundamental adjustment of the dis-ease picture, probably due to the use of the bowel nosode.

CASE 11.2   Vanity strikes back

A lady had exhibited concerns about her appearance for many years, result-
ing in cosmetic surgery on two occasions. Following the second operation a
benign lesion appeared in the region of the first intervention. The option of
further surgery to remove this lesion is rejected and the use of a bowel nosode
resolves the matter.

A thirty year old lady had been in a steady relationship for the past
five years when she presented with a firm enlargement on the upper
right side of her nose parallel to the inner canthus of the eye. This
had appeared first some two months prior to the homeopathic consultation and although it had grown slowly but steadily was none painful
either intrinsically or on palpation. It appeared roughly cone shaped,
approximately a quarter of an inch wide at its base and protruding
about half that at its highest point above the surface of the nose:
although it was not interfering with vision, the lady was aware
constantly of its presence. It was accompanied by a slight opaque
mucoid discharge from the right nostril, the only effect of which was
to cause her to blow her nose somewhat more frequently than normal.

Conventional help had been sought and an x-ray had been taken
along with a general examination. The x-ray showed an enlargement,
possibly with both bony and soft tissue involvement, protruding only
slightly into the nasal cavity, with its main volume being external.
No other physical abnormality had been found. Clinical assessment
did not considered that it was likely to be malignant. A course of antibiotics was prescribed (on general principles?) and the only other
advice offered had been to 'see how it goes' with the possibility of
surgical removal. Perhaps surprisingly in view of the lady's history,
this latter was not considered a desirable option and homeopathy had
been suggested (not by her doctor) as a route to be explored before
that extreme and when the antibiotics had produced no benefit she
acted on the suggestion.

She was an attractive lady with a lively personality. She worked as
the sales manager of a locally based company and enjoyed her job as
'it gave her the opportunity to put her ideas into practice'; she
admitted to being both a bad subordinate and an intolerant boss
when people did not match her enthusiasm and energy. Her early
medical history was unremarkable and included the usual vaccinations and acute illnesses of her childhood era. Apart from the nose

her only other medical problem was occasional migraine attacks which could on occasion be severe. During childhood she had been considered to be recklessly adventurous and still enjoyed high risk activities as a adult. After leaving school she had obtained a good degree in business studies as well as being involved fully in the sporting activities of her university. During her late teens she had developed a complex about the shape of her nose and finally cosmetic surgery had been undertaken, to her complete satisfaction. However, whilst at university she had become concerned about her weight, ostensibly to improve her sporting prowess. This developed into a major anorexic problem which persisted for some time beyond her time at university. Finally the acute situation resolved, apparently due to a combination of guidance and increasing satisfaction with her developing career, although she remained conscious of her weight and time at the gym became an integral part of her life style. After setting up home with her partner her devotion to the gym continued and in addition she developed a dissatisfaction with the size of her breasts, which she considered to be too small. Finally, she resorted to further surgery to 'correct' this, the procedure being considered a success by all concerned. It was some six months after this latest surgery that the presenting condition appeared.

The lady considered herself to be essentially 'normal'. There were no significant fears and her general approach to life was one of confidence in her ability to deal with any situation with which she might be confronted. When exercising she would always set herself specific targets. There was a sentimental side to her nature and she admitted enjoying a good cry when watching happy films, whilst genuine suffering or injustice made her angry. She liked to be comfortable with regard to heat but was happy to be out in the cold if it involved exercise. Her thirst was small but there was a liking for coffee; tea would be drunk occasionally but it had to be weak. In the main she avoided alcohol because she considered it to be fattening rather than there being any adverse taste or other health connotations for her. In many ways she showed a genuine indifference to food except for an evening glass of wine or two and an evening meal after a busy day. At other times she was content to 'graze' throughout the day with a mouthful here and there of whatever was available: her only positive desire was for chocolate.

An initial prescription of Bacillus No. 10 30c was made, with three doses to be taken in twenty four hours. The immediate and only effect was a change in the nature of the nasal discharge which became thicker to the extent of blocking the nostril, without any change in colour or volume. The left nostril did not become involved. This effect persisted for about a week and then eased with the discharge ceasing completely after ten days. One month after taking the remedy there had been only a slight increase in the size of the lesion and the right nostril remained discharge free. Bacillus No. 10 30c was repeated using the same twenty four hour regime as previously, this time with no major effect whatever except that the enlargement in the nose ceased completely. After another month the Bacillus No. 10 was repeated at 200c. Over the next three months there was a steady reduction in the nasal swelling and her conventional advisers, without offering any explanation, were content just to monitor the situation clinically. No further investigations were undertaken. During that time the lady suffered one severe attack of migraine but at the end all that remained was a small stable lump on the nose discernable only by those who knew what had been there before. A further single dose of Bacillus No. 10 200c was given and the lesion resolved completely. All has been clear for eighteen months since the last treatment and although the lady still suffers migraine attacks, her impression is that they are less frequent.

Discussion

The absence of an exact diagnosis in this case is, from the purist viewpoint, undesirable, but its clinical resolution without any major interference is obviously a preferable outcome. There are a number of remedies, such as Hecla Larva, Aurum Met and Symphytum that might have been considered in general terms based on the symptoms, although there was no over-whelming indication for any particular one. This situation provides one of the possible indications for the use of a bowel nosode, namely to clarify a symptom picture, and given the author's propensity to turn to bowel nosodes this was the route chosen. The personality and history of the patient pointed clearly to Bacillus No. 10 and as, from the evidence of the x-ray and the clinical opinion, this appeared to be a predominantly sycotic rather than a syphilitic reaction the physical symptoms fitted the remedy as well. As the initial dose had produced some reaction but no material change in the symptoms it was decided to persevere with the remedy as it was thought that it could be acting as a primary remedy rather than initiating any change in the presenting syndrome. In retrospect the decision to repeat the 30c potency could be considered a mistake and although the nasal enlargement had finally ceased an earlier increase in potency could have been a better option. Fortunately, in the event, the only loss was one of time. The significance, if any, of the migraine attack is difficult to gauge and could be irrelevant to the progress of the case. Certainly there have been further attacks since treatment ceased but any reliable assessment of their frequency and severity has not been forthcoming. The lady's lifestyle has not changed significantly although it is reported that her eating habits have become more consistent.

Whether the latest surgery acted as a trigger for the condition is speculative: no other aetiology was identified and it may be significant that the lesion appeared in the region of the initial intervention. In any event the bowel nosode appeared to act not only as a remedy in its own right but at a constitutional level.

12

THE SMALLER GROUPS
Mutabile, Faecalis, Coccal Co. and Poly Bowel

General considerations

'Smaller' in this context refers to both the frequency with which the respective NLFB have been found and also the number of associated remedies that have been identified with each of the bowel nosodes, and hence the narrower symptom picture that is available. The frequency with which the NLFB are found is less than with some of the other groups but, when indicated, the importance and effects of the appropriate bowel nosodes can be as great as with any of those more commonly used.

Materia medica

Mutabile

Traditionally associated remedies
Ferrum Phos, Kali Phos, Kali Sulph, **Pulsatilla Nig**.

Mutabile is so named because of the tendency of its associated bacteria to mutate immediately on culture from being non lactose to lactose fermenters. The nosode's theme of 'changeability' is mirrored in this. Mentally the picture is one of instability and capriciousness leading to insecurity and stress, as seen in its leading remedy, Pulsatilla. Mentally Pulsatilla exhibits a rapid changing of mood and opinions, and the type is easily swayed by the opinions of others, whilst on the physical level symptoms can be variable. Kali Sulph. is another of the associated remedies and this has many similarities to Pulsatilla in its remedy picture. It is the equivalent to Pulsatilla in the Schuesssler tissue salt range of medicines and it is interesting to note that potassium sulphate, its source material, is found in considerable quantity in the flowers of Pulsatilla (Morrison 1993).

The disease picture calling for the nosode will show an alternation of symptoms throughout the case history. This may take the form of the same symptom moving to different locations in the body but nevertheless staying within the same body system: pain in joints may move, for example, from elbow to knee to wrist to ankle and back again for no apparent reason, nor is the same laterality always maintained. Alternatively there may be a change of symptoms between systems, again for no obvious reason. In these situations, one of the systems involved is almost invariably the skin. One such condition is asthma where the lung symptoms alternate spontaneously with skin eruptions. Metastasis in cases of neoplasia is another possible indication under the same keynote. A sensitivity to suppressive treatments is another possible manifestation of the 'change-ability' characteristic.

The nosode has uses in urinary infections in general, particularly involving the bladder, and cases of recurrent and sub-acute cystitis can be helped (Paterson E 1960). These are accompanied by frequency and urgency but without intense pain in either bladder or urethra. Julian (1995) quotes Foubister as considering that albuminuria is an indication and Brown (1989) cites John Paterson himself using Mutabile as a 'near specific' in such cases. Some cases of malnutrition call for the nosode.

Miasmatically the balance is dominated by the sycotic influence as seen in Pulsatilla, reinforced by the Kali Sulph., which has both psoric and sycotic features. The psoric effect is added to by the Ferrum Phos., another associated remedy of the group. The overall balance is hence sycotic/psoric.

MUTABILE	
Mind	Capriciousness. Insecurity.
Urogenital	Urinary infections. Cystitis with frequency and urgency but no pain. Albuminuria.
Respiratory	Asthma alternating with skin symptoms.
Skin	Commonly involved with changeable symptoms in body.
Modalities & Generalities	Changeability on both mental and physical levels.

Faecalis

Traditionally associated remedy
Sepia Off.

Faecalis is one of the least used of the bowel nosodes; John Paterson found few clinical indications for it and only one remedy, namely Sepia, to be associated with it. The position of Anacardium in relation to the nosode and the resulting possibility of a keynote of 'duality' for it is discussed in Chapter 3. Two other remedies have also suggested as being associated, Thuja and Sulphur (Elliott 1996). Thuja would certainly fit into the theme that is proposed. The psychic dimension of the remedy has been vividly described by Coulter (1998), together with the battle against it that often goes on in the individual. The multi-faceted manifestations of the Sulphur nature may also be encompassed, although there is not necessarily the battle against the two sides of an individual's nature that is seen in the other quoted remedies. If this idea is correct, the key would appear to lie in the strength of the contradictory emotions that are involved in the remedy pictures. The 'duality' that is such a feature of the sycotic miasm (Lilley 2007; Saxton 2006) would be consistent with this interpretation as would the idea that mentally the type is driven by a desire for understanding of themselves and their situation (Malcolm 2007). The inclusion of Carcinosin as an associated remedy would also fit the pattern, and the dissociation and feeling of detachment from life that is found in the Carcinosin picture is could be regarded as an expression of this, along with the deep sense of dissatisfaction that is found in the remedy picture. Thus it will be seen that the remedy is now included in the Amended Associated Remedy List under Faecalis (see Appendix).

Mentally there is anger, either manifest or suppressed, and social considerations feature in the aetiology. These may be either a sensitivity to social pressures and a desire to conform (Carcinosin) or a failure to fit into a social situation as a result of a failure or inability to communication. Dissatisfaction with and loss of confidence in themselves may lead to a withdrawal into ordinary tasks with nothing original being attempted. The suppression of anger due to social pressures, with in some cases subsequent emotional explosion, as seen in the Staphisagria picture could indicate that remedy's inclusion among the associated remedies, but clinical experience has not yet confirmed this.

In the digestive sphere the nosode exhibits a particular susceptibility to inadequate diets. Processed foods will often upset patients and there is a marked upset from fats and all sugars, this latter being where its aggravation

FAECALIS	
Mind	Anger either expressed or suppressed. Sensitive to social situations. Lack of confidence in own performance.
Alimentary	Upset by fats and sugars. <sweets. Sensitive to inadequate diets and processed foods. Faeces like hard balls.

from sweets comes from. Stools may become like hard balls. Emotional changes will produce corresponding changes in bowel function.

Miasmatically the major influence is sycotic.

Coccal Co.

Traditionally associated remedies
Tuberculinum Bov.

The uses for this nosode appear to be linked primarily to septic states, although low- grade persistent infections will often also benefit. Such infections will not be of a systemic nature, rather being found in localised areas of the body, for example the low- grade infection that is found occasionally in the udder of a dairy cow. Such an indication is particularly relevant in view of the widespread presence of the tubercular miasm in cattle and the strong connection, via its associated remedies, of the nosode to that miasm. The skin may show pustular eruptions.

Within the context of Hahnemann's basic miasmatic concept, the tubercular miasm is widely regarded as a mixed miasm of psora and syphilis, although there is in fact a more significant sycotic influence than is sometimes supposed (Saxton 2006). The bowel nosode reflects this and the miasmatic balance in it is syphilitic/sycotic. The most commonly quoted indication in humans is in the treatment of boils and carbuncles.

Use of the nosode should be limited to very short courses in moderate potency. John Paterson specified a maximum of three doses only, using a 30c. Others have used 12c with success (Agrawal 1995). According to John Paterson the nosode should not be used in cases of diabetes mellitus, although no clear reason is given for this other than his experience. Equally, there is no indication as to whether this ban applies to all types of diabetes.

Poly Bowel

This is also known as 'Bach polyvalent nosode'. It is not a separate bowel nosode but rather a mixture of all the other nosodes except Sycotic Co. Its use as a clearing remedy was discussed in Chapter 4. Clinically it has also been used on the indication of 'rheumatism accompanied by constipation'. Whitmont regarded this as a leading indication for the mixture, using it at 200c. This is a particular example of a more general application where symptoms in a case are present in both the bowels and another system of the body concurrently. (It should be noted, however, that if the non bowel symptoms show clearly the theme of another of the bowel nosodes, it is often better to use that). Laing has used it with success in cases of chronic sinusitis (both quoted by Agrawal 1995) and its successful use as a cleansing remedy following antibiotics has been reported (Hunton 2010).

CASE 12.1   An outstanding symptom

One very strong symptom determines the choice of remedy, which is initially successful. Support from the associated bowel nosode does not resolve matters but moves the case's miasmatic expression, leading to a change of bowel nosode.

A three-and-a-half-year old entire male Springer spaniel was presented for homeopathic treatment after conventional treatment had failed to resolve recurrent attacks of abdominal colic. He had been bred by friends of the owners and weaned at six weeks of age, arriving in his present home at eight weeks old. There had been no problems with either whelping or rearing: contact had been maintained with one of the dog's litter mates, a female now neutered, and she had experienced no health problems. The mother also had no history of major health problems.

The dog had received his primary vaccinations at nine and twelve weeks of age, and a booster at twenty months old. Routine worming with a prescription agent had been carried out on both occasions. There had been no obvious reactions to any of the vaccinations, nor had there been any health problems other than the presenting colic.

The problem had started when he was three years old with a severe attack of colic followed by explosive diarrhoea. There had been no warning or obvious cause for the attack, but as it occurred over Christmas the owners assumed that it was in some way linked to the festivities and 'something he ate'. They had massaged his abdomen and the pain had passed quickly, while the motion was loose for twenty-four hours but without the initial explosiveness. Great care was subsequently taken over his diet, but in spite of this there was another episode five days later, and the attacks then became a regular occurrence. The onset was always sudden, there was never any vomiting or excessive flatulence, and once the pain had passed he would eat and drink normally. There had been no weight loss over the time the problem had been present and apart from the attacks the dog appeared perfectly normal.

Conventional veterinary help was sought, and treatment was commenced with oral steroids, betamethasone night and morning. There were no attacks whilst on that regime but they returned as soon as the dosage was reduced to once daily. Laboratory examination of the faeces revealed no abnormalities. The abdomen had been x-rayed, both with and without a barium meal, with nothing unusual being found. Standard blood screening had likewise shown complete normality. The owners had been advised that an exploratory laparotomy was the next investigative stage but they were unwilling to go down that route. They were also unhappy with the prospect of long-term steroids. The frequency of the attacks was consistent at around one a week, and as they had found that they could relieve the pain quickly by abdominal massage they had ceased treatment on their own volition. It was at this point that homeopathic help was requested.

At the homeopathic consultation the dog appeared perfectly normal. Abdominal palpation was not resented and no abnormality was detected. General physical also examination revealed no problems. He was a friendly dog, but after an initial greeting he returned to his owners, settled at their feet, and 'napped'. However, at the mention of his name, he lifted his head immediately and looked around, but did not move from near his owners. He was said to be friendly with all dogs and people. If another dog appeared in any way aggressive he would growl slightly and back away. Adult visitors to the house were initially greeted with enthusiasm and then ignored. There were two children in the household and when they had friends round the dog would want to be involved in their activities. He had no particular favourites among the family, did not follow any of them around, and was happy to be on his own. He had never caused any damage in the house. There were no other animals in the family.

He had no marked fears and was unmoved by thunder. He hated the vacuum cleaner and would bark all the time it was in use if he was anywhere near it. He appeared neutral about heat in the house but enjoyed lying out in the sun. He was happy to go out for a walk in any weather that the owners were prepared to go out in, and would go outside on his own for toilet purposes in any conditions.

His appetite and thirst were described as normal, and neither of these had changed whilst he had been on steroids. He was fed on proprietary tinned food and biscuit supplemented by scraps. There had never been any undue flatulence. Motions were normal except when associated with a colic attack and at such times the diarrhoea contained a moderate amount of mucus, but never any blood.

When he had an attack he would go very quiet suddenly and start to whimper. He would assume the 'prayer position', with his head and elbows on the ground, his hind quarters up in the air and his spine arched ventrally; if left alone he would remain in that pose. During the initial attacks, the owners had thought that it was the massage they applied to the abdomen that relieved the situation. However, they had come to realise that all that was necessary to give relief was the proximity of one of them and the giving of sympathy to the dog. Accordingly, in the event of an attack, they had now adopted the routine of lifting him onto a knee, stroking his head and talking in a sympathetic manner. After one to two minutes of this the dog would jump down and proceed as if nothing had happened.

The only indication of a time modality was the fact that there had never been an attack at night, nor was there any obvious physical or emotional trigger. The last episode had occurred four days prior to the consultation.

Pulsatilla 30c night and morning for four days was prescribed. A telephone call two weeks later reported that there had been no further attacks and the dog appeared normal in every way. Following that, all remained well for four months.

After that time the dog was re-presented having developed an irritation down the length of his back and a sore on his left shoulder. There were no other lesions, no dandruff, and the whole coat felt dry. The irritation had started some ten days previously for no apparent reason, but the colic attacks had not returned. The owners felt that the dog wanted more attention and the scratching could be stopped by giving it, but he was otherwise still normal. A systemic flea treatment (although no fleas had been found) and steroids had been prescribed by the referring vet but the latter had not been given.

The prescription of Pulsatilla was repeated as before. This stopped the irritation and the sore healed in around one week, but the problem returned after another three weeks, this time accompanied by an attack of colic. Sympathy alone resolved this as before. The potency of Pulsatilla was increased to 200c and given night and morning for three days. This gave no improvement and so after one month Mutabile 30c was administered night and morning for three days. There was one moderately severe attack of colic two days after finishing the course but no more since. However, the skin had worsened over the next three weeks, being still irritant and developing some red patches without heat. Sores with a thin watery discharge had appeared behind both knees (wrists). The dog was still eating well and happy in himself.

At this point Morgan Bach 30c was administered night and morning for four days. After two weeks there had been no further bowel problems and the skin had improved by, on the owner's estimation, about 60%. The improvement had, however, ceased but not regressed. The Morgan Bach was repeated at 200c night and morning for two days, after which all symptoms disappeared. The dog has remained normal ever since.

Discussion

At the initial consultation, the problem was clearly presenting as a sycotic manifestation, with the colic involving the 'prayer position' and the explosive diarrhoea followed by mucus in the stool. There were certain pointers towards Pulsatilla in the dog's case history, such as the submissive tendency and the friendliness. Another clue, in the author's experience, was the lack of increased thirst whilst on steroids, almost a form of 'thirstlessness'. However, the overriding feature was the marked amelioration from sympathy, and this was the deciding factor in the selection of the remedy. The initial success confirmed the choice. However, the subsequent development of a skin aspect changed the perception of the case. With hindsight it might have been better to have changed the prescription at the first appearance of the skin symptoms, but it was felt at the time that the previous success of the Pulsatilla plus the still strong influence of sympathy present justified persisting with the approach. Its subsequent limited effect dictated a change of remedy. The Mutabile had the effect of clearing the presenting picture by emphasising the skin dimension of the case. The choice of Morgan Bach was due to the author's devotion to bowel nosodes and in this situation others may have chosen Sulphur or some other predominantly anti-psoric remedy instead. In the event the remedy chosen was successful. It is interesting to speculate as to which of the nosodes, the Mutabile or the Morgan Bach, finally resolved the abdominal symptom. The symptoms are more reflected in the Morgan Bach remedy picture but the success of the Pulsatilla may point to some influence from the Mutabile. Both Mutabile and Morgan Bach have sycotic connections that fit the overall pattern of this case.

In some ways this case mirrors the case of John Paterson's discussed in Chapter 2, where the appropriate bowel nosode changed with the symptoms as the case progressed. This emphasises once more that the principles governing the use of the bowel nosodes are common to both humans and animals.

CASE 12.2   A victim of circumstances

A cat is involved in a territorial dispute and as a result develops a problem of persistent infection. The initial remedy fails to act but the bowel nosodes opens up the case.

A seven-year-old neutered female domestic shorthair cat had fallen victim to the bullying activities of a semi-feral tomcat that had moved into the area around her home. As is the way of such visitors, the tomcat had remained in the area for some two months and had then moved on. However, during that time he had employed the usual tactic of pouncing on his victims from behind and had consequently inflicted a series of bites around the hindquarters of the innocent female. She, being at first unsuspecting, had initially sustained two or three severe bites around the pelvic area and into the large muscle groups on the posterior of the hind legs. Similarly the owner, being equally unsuspecting, had failed to appreciate the significance of the sudden onset hind leg lameness in her cat, with the result that a large deep seated abscess had been allowed to develop. It was only when this abscess burst that the full extent of the problem was realised and treatment sought. This, from a conventional colleague, consisted of antibiotic cover accompanied by flushing and draining, facilitated by in-patient care and daily injections of Synulox (clavulanic acid and amoxycillin) for five days. This appeared to resolve the situation, but unfortunately the cat was attacked again shortly after her return home, sustaining another bite in the same region. There were now reports from other owners in the area of similar events involving their animals. The root cause of the problem being realised, antibiotic treatment was instigated immediately by means of oral Baytril (enrofloxacin) once daily for ten days, and another major abscess was avoided.

In spite of these experiences the cat still continued to go outside, although she became more wary. As a result several more bites were sustained over about a month, although the attacks were both less frequent and severe. As far as was known, antibiotics were given on every occasion.

The tomcat finally moved on as evidenced by the cessation of the attacks. However, the cat continued to have problems, with periodic hind leg lameness accompanied by some breakdown of the apparently healed abscesses. The resulting fistulae produced on occasion both serous and pustular discharges. Although continuing to eat reasonably well the cat lost some weight and general condition. Courses of various antibiotics were used, plus injections of anabolic steroid (Nandrolin), but without success, and the cat was passed to a colleague within the same practice for homeopathic treatment. The owner had added Echinacae herbal drops to the treatment on her own initiative.

The cat was of average build and described as 'friendly yet independent'. She had free access via a cat flap, and before the troubles started she would spend most of her time outside, mainly in and around her own garden but sometimes venturing further afield. She had never been known to stay out all night. She would stay out in rain but did not like cold, although when she came in she would never seek a source of heat. She was not thought of as a nervous cat. Appetite was described as generally normal but thirst could not be accurately ascertained due to the time she spent outside. The occasional mouse was brought in dead as an 'offering', but she did not appear as a voracious hunter. She was not going out as much as normal but this was thought to be due to the current problem. The area around the hindquarters was not unduly sensitive to touch, and there was no aggressive reaction to palpation of the area. She would move around the house and garden but her owner described her movements as 'slower than normal'. She had been seen to jump. Rectal temperature was normal at the consultation. Mucous membrane colour was good. Heart and lungs were normal on auscultation and there was no noticeable abnormality in the temperature of the hind legs.

Silica 30c was chosen as the treatment and administered night and morning for five days as an essentially local prescription. There was not the sensitivity or anger that might indicate Hepar Sulph., that being the main remedy considered as an alternative. In spite of warning the owner of the possibility of increased discharges this did not happen to any marked degree. Re-examination two weeks later showed no change.

Coccal Co. 30c was then prescribed, three doses over a twenty-four hour period. Within a week the cat appeared brighter in herself and the appetite was improving although there was no great physical change. After another week there was definitely less discharge from the sinuses. However, a marked degree of sensitivity had developed over the affected region. Hepar Sulph. 200c night and morning for three days was given, and this led to the complete resolution of the problem.

Discussion

It is clear that a low-grade persistent infection was present in this case, but the interesting aspect was the emergence, after the administration of the Coccal Co, of the indication for a remedy that had been rejected previously as not fitting the presenting picture in any way, and the success following the use of the Hepar Sulph. The Coccal Co. was prescribed as a remedy in its own right, whereas in fact it appeared to act in a different way. The choice of potency with Hepar Sulph. being between the high to abort suppuration as opposed to the low to encourage it, it was felt that what was being seen was in many ways a 'never well since' situation. Although the first abscess had run its natural course, the subsequent use of antibiotics for the later infections had acted as a form of suppression. Hepar Sulph. does not appear to have been linked to Coccal Co. in the past. and although it is possible that Hepar Sulph. should be considered as another associated remedy, the evidence of one case is insufficient to establish that beyond question. Alternatively the effect of the Coccal Co. could be interpreted as moving the case towards cure rather than merely accentuating the clarity and activity of an associated remedy.

CASE 12.3 A persistent nuisance

A middle aged man is left with a recurring sore throat following a severe winter cold/flue. Other remedies help with the acute phase but a bowel nosode is used to resolve the throat.

A sixty-two year-old man had suffered from an infection beginning towards the end of November. At first this appeared to be no more than just a winter cold, displaying a clear watery bilateral nasal discharge accompanied by sneezing and a feeling of mild fullness in the frontal and nasal regions of the head. However, within two days there had been a marked worsening. The feeling of fullness had increased and his eyes had begun to ache. In spite of the nasal discharge, the nose felt blocked and could not be cleared by blowing, although this was productive. The sneezing continued and a sore throat and moist cough appeared. There was a systemic lassitude with aching in all muscles. The abdomen was described as 'uncomfortable', and looseness of the bowels developed, although there was no frank diarrhoea or vomiting. The nasal discharge became thicker, although still clear, and mucus appeared in the back of the throat. Expectoration was easy but did not relieve. There was no difficulty swallowing. Appetite was reduced but thirst remained normal.

There was no history of any susceptibility to colds. Apart from an increasing degree of stiffness in the lumbar region associated with a prolapsed spinal disc of around twenty years standing, there was no significant medical history. He had enjoyed good health all his life, which he took for granted. His life style was active, involving walking and recreational swimming; no formal sport was now undertaken. He was essentially tidy and organised, and liked to plan in advance. Travel was enjoyed when it was necessary, as it was periodically with his job, but he would never travel just for the sake of the experience. Holidays were selected primarily on the basis of revisiting places enjoyed previously. One of his main criterion was that the location was not too crowded, although complete solitude was equally un-desirable. Almost invariably he enjoyed new experiences although initially reluctant to venture into them. His taste in food was similarly conservative. In addition to a genuine dislike of spices, and an almost pathological hatred of garlic and salt, he was unwilling to try new things on principle. For reasons of taste he would not normally eat butter or cream unless presented with them in a 'social' situation. He was keen on salads, vegetables and fruits other than citrus. He could be indifferent to food but his appetite was large if he started to eat. Thirst was described as 'average'; if a drink was designed to be hot then it had to be very hot, and he could drink it quickly. Conversely, cold drinks were also enjoyed, and he disliked food that was too hot in temperature. Bowels were normal and there was no tendency to flatulence. He had a slight preference for warmth rather than cold, but only became distressed in extreme cold. He was happy to go out in all weathers except severe wind.

As soon as the initial symptoms had appeared, Echinacea 825mgm once daily had been taken, and this was continued. When the condition worsened, a sequence of three remedies, Arsenicum Iod., Gelsemium and Eupatorium Perf. was taken at a 30c potency night and morning for three days. This treatment was selected on general principles as having shown to be effective in cases displaying general 'flue' type symptoms (Brown quoting John Paterson). By the fourth day all symptoms had disappeared except for a degree of mucus around the throat and nasal passages. This continued to improve for the next week until all that was left was some slight nasal congestion, but then the sore throat returned.

At this stage the throat presented as definitely on the right side. There was no difficulty in swallowing and both eating and drinking relieved the soreness temporarily. A dry cough developed due to an intermittent tickling on the hard palate and a feeling of fullness in the throat. A dull pain appeared extending from the throat to the ear, exactly where he was unable to identify. There was no aural discharge. No systemic symptoms returned.

The Echinacea was continued with, and Lycopodium 30c was administered night and morning for three days. This was selected primarily because of the right sidedness, the increased mucus, the general features of liking very hot drinks with the ability to drink them and the large appetite once stimulated. The remedy produced an easing of around 50% but did not clear the problem. After a week Lycopodium 200c was given night and morning for three doses. This gave no additional benefit although the initial improvement was maintained. The immediate thought was to move to Morgan Gaertner as the bowel nosode primarily associated with Lycopodium. However, at this stage the patient accompanied members of his family on a short skiing holiday, solely as an (albeit reluctant) observer. Whilst at the alpine resort the throat cleared completely, but shortly after his return it re-appeared with the additional symptom of a malodorous mouth. There was no pain from the teeth or sign of ulceration in the mouth. The only sign was a slight inflammation of the right tonsil. Cervical lymph nodes were not enlarged and there was no reaction to palpation of the throat.

It was concluded that there was still a low grade infection present in the throat, and accordingly Coccal Co. 30c night and morning for three doses was prescribed. Within twenty-four hours all symptoms began to subside, and after four days had completely disappeared. After ten days some slight mucus re-appeared in the throat and a very slight feeling of discomfort recurred up towards the right ear. A single dose of Coccal Co. 200c was given and all was resolved after three days. There was no return of the condition.

Discussion

The Coccal Co. in this case was used as a remedy in its own right, based on an essentially pathological prescription. The initial use of Lycopodium seemed indicated not only by the local symptoms but also by aspects of the patient's personality. The only remedy traditionally associated with Coccal Co. is Tuberculinum, which did not appear to fit the patient. However, it is interesting to note the aspect of his character that ended up enjoying new experiences. Also, Lycopodium is regarded by many as having a tubercular connection (Banerjea 2003), and it is interesting to speculate as to the possible significance of this. The idea of using Morgan Gaertner was not pursued as the symptom picture had changed after the return from the Alps. Hepar Sulph., and especially Gunpowder, are two remedies that are often of use in similar circumstances of infection, but neither seemed appropriate in this case. Of the sequence of remedies given originally, Gelsemium appeared to have the closest overall fit to the symptom picture, including sore throat with pain extending into the ear, but some features of the picture are found in the other two remedies.

CASE 12.4   Overcoming a conventional block

The solution to a chronic problem appears clear but the indicated treatment produces no effect. The reason lies in the prior conventional treatment and once that is overcome the indicated remedies produce the desired effect.

An eight year old black and white neutered male domestic shorthair cat had suffered from an intermittent bilateral nasal discharge for four years. He had lived with the same lady in the same house all his life, having been found with two litter mates as a stray kitten of around six or seven weeks of age. Although in poor condition when found, all had appeared basically healthy; his litter mates had been re-homed and he had been reared with no significant health problems. He had been neutered, wormed and vaccinated against 'flue and enteritis as a kitten (exact dates unknown) and had subsequently been wormed and received regular boosters at approximately yearly intervals without any recorded ill effects. There was one other cat in the household, a neutered female around a year older who had been there when the kitten arrived. He had been completely subservient to her all his life. Neither cat had suffered any major health problems apart from the resenting complaint in the male, which had never affected the female.

The male's problem had started in June four years previously for no obvious reason. The first sign had been mild sneezing followed by a pale, whitish mucoid bilateral nasal discharge. The cat remained lively with his appetite unimpaired. A course of antibiotic (Ceporex) produced no dramatic improvement but the condition slowly improved and resolved in, as far as could be remembered, about two weeks. There had been another attack in the October which had followed a similar course. The pattern continued over the next three years, gradually worsening with the attacks becoming more frequent and the discharge becoming thicker, although not purulent. Booster vaccinations continued to be given with no marked connection to the attacks. Various antibiotics had been used, all with limited success although culture of the discharge had shown bacterial sensitivity to the antibiotics. The skull had been x-rayed but no gross abnormality had been found. By the time homeopathic help was sought the attacks were happening frequently with only short breaks between them. On occasion the sneezing contained small amounts of fresh blood. The cat was less lively and had lost some appetite. Repeated courses of antibiotics had been administered to minimal effect.

Homeopathic consultation

Although there had been some weight loss the general condition was still adequate. No vomiting or diarrhoea had been seen. There was no pain on palpation of the nasal and frontal region The appetite was described as 'poor', no vomiting had been observed and as far as was known the motions were normal. It was impossible to form an accurate assessment of his thirst as there was a communal supply, but the impression was that there was no great thirst. The chest was clear on auscultation and abdominal palpation revealed no abnormality. All examinations were well tolerated with no dissent. The lady confirming the cat's easy going temperament and the fact that she had always been able to do anything with him. Her only complaint about him was that he was a fierce hunter who regularly deposited dead mice in the house in spite of her expressed disapproval. He was initially cautious of strangers but quickly overcame that and then sought attention from them. The cat would lie out in the sun for a while but indoors avoided radiators. Once settled on anyone's knee he would remain there although panting.

A three-day course of Pulsatilla 30c b d was prescribed, which produced a slight temporary brightening but no change in either appetite or discharge. Three days of Pulsatilla 200C b d had the same effect. A potency chord (6,30,200c) of Mutabile o d for three days was followed by a repeat of the Pulsatilla 30c without producing the desired effect. After further consideration of the history a chord (6, 30,200) of Polybowel o d for three days, the only observed effect being an increase in the sneezing. Ten days after the course ended Pulsatilla 30c b d three days was again administered. This time the cat brightened considerably and the appetite improved although the nasal discharge increased. The improvement ceased before was the condition had cleared but was maintained. Two further courses of Pulsatilla 30c finally resolved the problem.

Discussion

With hindsight the Polybowel could have been given earlier but the indication for the particular remedy was so clear that it was persevered with. It is worth noting that the cat was still a keen and successful hunter in spite of his constitutional type, and this is normal. He might, as the lady said, 'never hurt a fly' but instinct ensured that mice were not included in the general amnesty and the fact of the regular presentation of his trophies could in part be attention seeking, a trait that the lady inadvertently encouraged by giving him attention. When the initial Pulsatilla failed to act a change to Silica was considered but rejected in favour of an increased potency. Similarly Gaertner Bach was considered in view of the antibiotic overload but rejected due to its remedy and miasmatic connections.

APPENDIX

The expanded associated remedy lists

The following lists must be regarded as being to some degree more speculative than the traditional original lists presented in Chapter 2 and represent a broader clinical experience than is quoted there. Those early lists represent the original remedies that were accepted as being linked to the respective bowel nosodes. In most cases that link had been established by both clinical observation and accompanying bacteriology.

However, during subsequent clinical use of the bowel nosodes, experience has shown other remedies to be linked. Because the role of the faecal swab in the clinical situation has, for practical purposes, ceased, later additions to the lists are based on observations in practice. The range of remedies being employed has also widened, both as a result of changing clinical patterns over the years and the introduction of new remedies. The following lists contain all those remedies in addition to the commonly agreed members, and represent the thoughts and clinical observations of all the major workers in the field, plus the clinical experience of other practitioners. Thus John Paterson's thoughts about various remedies which were not included in the original lists are quoted here, and Anacardium has been added as linked to Faecalis based on the experience of the author and other veterinary colleagues. Similarly increased clinical experience may necessitate changes to the grading of some individual remedies.

Morgan Pure

Alumina, Antimony Crudum, Baryta Carbonicum, Calcarea Carbonicum, Calcarea Fluorica, Calcarea Silicata, Calcarea Sulphurica, Carbo Animalis, Carbo Vegetabilis, Causticum, Digitalis, Ferrum Carbonicum, *Graphites*, Gunpowder, Hamamelis, *Histamine*, Hepar Sulphuris, Kali Bichromicum, Kali Carbonicum, Kali Sulphuricum, Lac Humanum, Lycopodium Clavatum, Magnesia Carbonica, *Medorrhinum*, Natrum Carbonicum, Natrum

Sulphuricum, Nux Vomica, Petroleum, *Psorinum*, Pulsatilla, Rhus Toxico-dendron, Robinia, *Sepia Officinalis*, Silica, 'SSC', **Sulphur**, Thuja Occidentalis, Tuberculinum Bovinum.

Morgan Gaertner

Berberis Vulgaris, Calcarea Carbonica, Carbo Vegetabilis, Causticum, Chelidonium Majus, Chenopodium Anthelminticum, Graphites, Helleborus Niger, Hepar Sulphuris, Kali Bichromicum, *Lachesis Muta*, **Lycopodium Clavatum**, Mercurius Sulphuricus, Natrum Muriaticum, Nux Vomica, Pulsatilla, Sanguinaria Canadensis, Sarsaparilla, Sepia Officinalis, Silica, Sulphur, Taraxicum Officinalis.

Proteus

Ammonium Bromatum, Ammonium Muriaticum, Apis Mellifica, Aurum Muriaticum, Baryta Muriaticum, Borax, Calcarea Muriatica, Cholesterin, Colocynthis, Conium Maculatum, Cuprum Metallicum, Ferrum Muriaticum, Hepar Sulphuris, Hyoscyamus, *Ignatia Amara*, Kali Muriaticum, Magnesia Muriatica, Muriaticum Acidum, **Natrum Muriaticum**, Nitricum Acidum, Nux Vomica, Sarracenia Purpurea, Secale Cornutum, Sepia Officinalis, Staphysagria.

Mutabile

Camphor, Cimicifuga Racemosa, Ferrum Phosphoricum, Kali Phosphoricum, Kali Sulphuricum, Medorrhinum, **Pulsatilla**.

Gaertner Bach

Abrotanum, Aloe, Anacardium Orientale, Argentum Nitricum, Arsenicum Album, Bacillinum, Cadmium Metallicum, Calcarea Fluorica, Calcarea Hypophosphorosa, Calcarea Iodata, Calcarea Phosphorica, Calcarea Silicata, *Carcinosin*, Ferrum Phosphoricum, Kali Phosphoricum, Kalmia Latifolia, **Mercurius solubilis**, Natrum Fluoricum, Natrum phosphoricum, Natrum Silicatum, **Phosphorus**, Phosphoricum Acidum, Phytolacca, Podophyllum, Pulsatilla, Sanicula Aqua, **Silica**, Stannum Metallicum, *Syphilinum*, Tuberculinum*, Zincum Phosphoricum.

Dysentery Co.

Ammonium Carbonicum, Anacardium Orientale, Abies Canadensis, Abies Nigra, Antimony Crudum, *Argenticum Nitricum*, Arnica Montana, **Arsenicum Album**, Arsenicum Sulphuratum**, Bacillinum, Cactus Grandiflora, Carbo Vegetabilis, Carcinosin, China Arsenicosum, China Officinalis, Coffea Cruda, Digitalis, Dulcamara, Gelsemium Sempervirens, Graphites, Kali Arsenicum, Kali Carbonicum, **Kalmia Latifolia**, Kreosotum, Lachesis Muta, Lathyrus Sativus, Ledum Palustre, Lycopodium Clavatum, Magnesia Muriatica, Natrum Carbonicum, Phosphorus, Platina, Ptelea Trifoliata, Pulsatilla, Sanguinaria, Sarsaparilla, Sepia Officinalis, Spongia Tosta, Tuberculinum Bovinum, Veratrum Album, Veratrum Viride.

Bacillus No. 7

Arsenicum Iodatum, *Bromium*, Bryonia Alba, Calcarea Carbonica, Calcarea Fluorica, Calcarea Hypophosphorosa, Calcarea Iodatum, Carbo Vegetabilis, Causticum, Ferrum Iodatum, **Iodum**, Kali Bichromicum, Kali Bromatum, **Kali Carbonicum**, *Kali Iodatum*, Kali Nitricum, Mandragoria Officinarum, Mercurius Iodatum**, Natrum Iodatum, Rhus Toxicodendron, Sepia Officinalis, The 'acid remedies' generally.

Faecalis

Anacardium Orientale, Carcinosin, **Sepia Officinalis**.

Sycotic Co.

Antimonium Tartaricum, Bacillinum, Calcarea Carbonica, Calcarea Phosphorica, Antimonium Crudum, Calcium Metallicum***, Dulcamara, Ferrum Metallicum, Kali Bichromicum (consider the 'Kalis' generally), Lycopodium Clavatum, Medorrhinum, Morbillinum, Natrum Sulphuricum, Natrum Muriaticum, Nitricum Acidum, Pulsatilla, Rhus Toxicodendron, Sepia Officinalis, Silica, Sulphur, Tellurium, *Thuja Occidentalis,* Tuberculinum*.

Bacillus No. 10

Aralia Racemosa, Borax, *Calcarea Fluorica*, Calcarea Phosphorica, Hydrastis, Kali Bichromicum, Lachesis Muta, Medorrhinum, *Natrum Sulphuricum,*

Nitricum Acidum, Phosphorus, Platinum, Sabal Serrulata, Sepia Officinalis, Thuja Occidentalis.

Coccal Co.

Bacillinum, Hepar Sulphuris, *Tuberculinum**.

No growth

Bacllinum,Mercurius solubilis, Tuberculinum*.

Potency chords

The concept of potency chords, also known as 'potency complexes', was developed in the first half of the 20th century (Pedalino 2006). The technique involves the combination of two or more different potencies of the same remedy, prepared individually, in the same dose (Frase W 1999; Swayne 2000). The choice of the potency range selected will depend on its starting point, and the chord will then follow ascending potency steps. Clinically, these steps are generally determined by the concept of potency 'octaves' as commonly utilised in homeopathic prescribing. Thus a starting potency of 6c would then follow the sequence of 30c, 200c, 1M, 10M and on to CM: an alternative initial potency, such as 12x, would lead to a chord of a different range. As the name implies, the result has similarities to a musical chord, where sounds of a different pitch are combined. Medically, a remedy thus prepared will span the disease process more broadly that is possible with a single potency. Commonly, three individual potencies are used for a chord, although this number is variable depending on the wishes of the prescriber. The individual dose thus created may then be used in whatever dosage regime is deemed appropriate in a particular case.

The effect of giving a potency chord is not the same as using sequential doses of ascending potencies. There is an interaction between the potencies when administered as a chord that is not found with individual doses. One description of this process is that 'low potencies would have their effect on structures. . . . Intermediate potencies would have a regulatory effect on function. . . . High potencies would have the effect of information on the particular system' (Pedalino 2006). An alternative view favoured by the author is that the potency range offered allows the body to select the potency it requires for an exact energetic resonance between disease and remedy at any particular time. Subsequent doses will automatically allow for any slight alteration in the potency required by the body. (In Paragraphs 30–33 and 246–247 of the *Organon,* Hahnemann discusses the importance of the ability to adjust the medicinal energy of the similar medicine in order to achieve a curative process without increasing the possibility of aggravation.) Another idea that has been suggested is that 200c is not in fact the correct continuation of the sequence 6c>30c> but that it should be 125c (Dupree & Beal 2000) and if this is correct then the appropriate potency chord extending to 200c will cover that possibility.

Experimentally, potency chords have been found to produce less and milder aggravations than single potencies (Gomez 1992 quoted by Pedalino). Julian, in both his *Traite de micro-immunotherapie dynamisee* (1977) and *Materia medica der Nosoden* (1983), reports on his use of nosodes in potency chords and concludes that they are able to 'act more rapidly, deeply and lastingly and present fewer side effects' than other preparations (Pedalino 2006). (For these works Julian describes nosodes as 'biotherapeutic substances', and defines them as 'medicinal preparations obtained from microbial products, excretions and secretions whether pathological or otherwise – which definition would include bowel nosodes). It is also consistent with Kent's view of the correct remedy being merely what he calls the 'curative agent' whilst the 'simillimum' is that curative agent in the correct potency.

Potency chords allow a remedy to act to its deepest level, thus producing a true and lasting effect. Bowel nosodes are remedies that address the underlying upsets in 'dis-ease', and hence, in the author's view, lend themselves naturally to being used as potency chords. Over the years the author's clinical experience has made him change his prescribing regime when using potency chords from the single divided dose of three doses in twenty-four hours to one dose daily for three days.

Notes

* Although not always stated, Tuberculinum is generally considered to be Tuberculinum Bovinum. It is described as such in John Paterson's original list in relation to Morgan Pure.
** In the literature the exact form of Merc Iod used is unfortunately unclear. It may be that both forms are included. The same situation pertains to the entry for Arsenicum Sulphuratum.
*** See Chapter 2.

REFERENCES

Agrawal Y R (1995). *A Treatise on Bowel Nosodes*. New Delhi: Vijay Publications.

Alexander M (1988). Re-identifying the Bowel Nosodes. *British Homeopathic Journal*; **77**(2): 67–71.

Armstrong S E (2007). *Dynamic Groups – the Homeopathic Management of a Racing Yard*. BAHVS annual conference. Leeds.

Armstrong S E (2011). *Personal communication*.

Asher E (2006). *The delusion of the core delusion: was Richard Hughes really right? Removing obstacles to cure*. Proceedings of British Homeopathic Congress. Edinburgh, November 2006.

Asher E (2007). Removing Obstacles to Cure. *Simile (Faculty of Homeopathy newsletter)*; January.

Bach E (1920). The Relation of Vaccine Therapy to Homoeopathy. *British Homeopathic Journal*; **10**: 68–77.

Bach E (1922). The Confirmation of Homoeopathy by Modern Pathological Science. *British Homeopathic Journal*; **12**: 363–367.

Bach E (1928). An Effective Method of Combating Intestinal Toxaemia. *Medical World*; March 30th; 88–94.

Bach E (1929). The Rediscovery of Psora. *British Homeopathic Journal*; **19**: 29–50.

Bach E (1952). *The Twelve Healers and other Remedies*. 2nd edition (Revised). Saffron Walden, UK: C W Daniels.

Bach E & Wheeler C E (1925). *Chronic Disease a Working Hypothesis* London: H K Lewis. (Reprinted (1987); New Delhi: B Jain Publishers.)

Ball S (1996). *Flower Remedies a complete guide*. Leicester: Bookmark Ltd.

Banerjee S K (2003). *Miasmatic Diagnosis*. New Delhi: B Jain Publishers.

Blasig T, Vint P (2001). *Remedy Relationships*. Translated by Edmonds P, Waldbaum H. Greifenberg, D: Hahnemann Institut.

Boyd H (1989). *Introduction to Homeopathic Medicine*. 2nd ed. Beaconsfield: Beaconsfield Publishers.

Brown G (1967). Drs John and Elizabeth Paterson. *British Homeopathic Journal*; **56**: 201–218.

Brown G (1989). Drs John and Elizabeth Paterson: Reflections and Reminiscences. *The Homoeopath*; **8**(4): 3–14.

Bouhnik Y (1992). Fecal recovery in humans of viable Bifidobacterium sp. ingested in fermented milk. *Gastroenterology*; **102**: 857–878.

Bouhnik Y (1992). Fecal recovery in humans of viable Bifidobacterium sp. ingested in fermented milk. *Gastroenterology*; **102**: 857–878.

Carr A P (2007). New Approaches to Canine Epilepsy: Review of 23rd forum of the American College of Veterinary Internal Medicine. *Veterinary Times*; **37**: 22,26.

Chancellor P M (1971). *Handbook of the Bach Flower Remedies*. Saffron Walden, UK: C W Daniels. (Reprint 1985.)

Clarke J H (1982). *Dictionary of Practical Materia Medica*. Saffron Walden, UK: Health Science Press.

Coulter C R (1986). *Portraits of Homoeopathic Medicines* (Volume 1). Berkeley, CA: North Atlantic Books.

Coulter C R (1988). *Portraits of Homoeopathic Medicines* (Volume 2). Berkeley, CA: North Atlantic Books.

Coulter C R (1998). *Portraits of Homoeopathic Medicines* (Volume 3). Berkeley, CA: North Atlantic Books.

Cummings S (1988). History and Development of the Bowel Nosodes. *British Homeopathic Journal*; **77**: 72–77.

Dantas F, Fisher P, Walach H *et al* (2007). A systematic review of the quality of homeopathic pathogenetic trials published from 1945 to 1995. *Homeopathy*; **96**: 4–16.

Desrochers A M *et al* (2005). Efficacy of Saccharomyces boulardii for treatment of horses with acute enterocolitis. *Journal Am Vet Med Assoc*; **227**: 954–959.

Dishington T M (1927). The Autogenous Vaccines and their relation to Chronic Disease. *Transactions of International Homoeopathic Congress*. London.

Dishington T M (1929). The Pathogenesis of Dysentry and the Proving of the Nosode Dys Co. *British Homeopathic Journal*; **19**: 171–190.

Dorland (1974). *Illustrated Medical Dictionary*. 25th edn. London: W B Saunders.

Dukes H H (1955). *The Physiology of Domestic Animals*. 7th edn. London: Bailliere, Tindall & Cox.

Dupree G & Beal S (2000). *Rethinking Kent's Octaves*. BAHVS conference.

Elliott M F (1993). The role of Bowel Nosodes in the treatment of Disease. *BAHVS Conference Proceedings*. Durham, UK.

Elliott M F (1996). *Personal communication*.

Feldman M (1996). *A Repertory of the Bowel Nosodes*. New Delhi: B Jain Publishers.

Frase W (1999). La eficacia de las dilucions homeopatica en forma de acordes de potencia. *Medica Biologica. International Journal for Biomedical Research and Therapy*; **12**(2): 59–61.

Foubister D M (1988). Vomiting in infancy and childhood. *British Homeopathic Journal*; **77**: 117–123. (Reprint of original article published 1952.)

Fraefel D (2013). Narayana 2nd Veterinary Congress. April. Germany.

Fuller R (1989). Probiotics in man and animals. *J Appl Bacteriol*; **66**: 365–378.

Gomez J M (1992). Aportacion al estudio de la eficacia de la diluciones homeopaticas de Phosphorus. *Medica Biologica*; **1**: 4–14.

Gordon Ross (1973). The Bowel Nosodes. *British Homeopathic Journal*; **62**: 42–45.

Gregory P A (2000). *Personal communication*.

Hahnemann C F S (1796). Essay on a New Principle for Ascertaining the Curative Power of Drugs. *Lesser Writings* ed R E Dudgeon. (Reprinted 1933.) New Delhi: B Jain Publishers.

Hahnemann C F S (1830). *Materia Medica Pura*. New Delhi: B Jain Publishers.

Hahnemann C F S (1835). *The Chronic Diseases. Their Peculiar Nature and Their Homeopathic Cure*. Translated L H Tafel 1896 from the 2nd edn. (Reprinted 1978.) New Delhi: B Jain Publishers.

Hahnemann C F S (1921). *Organon of the Medical Art*. 6th ed. Decker S (trans.), Brewster O'Reilly (ed.) (1996). Redmont CA: Birdcage Books.

Hill D R, Artis D (2010). Intestinal bacteria and the regulation of immune cell homeostais: *Annual Review immunology*; **28**: 622–667.

Hunton M (2010). Nosodes in Clinical practice. *Faculty of Homeopathy Congress*, Cambridge, UK.

Hunton M (2010). *Personal communication*.

Julian O A (1977). *Traite de micro-immunotherapie dynamisee. Matiere Medicale des Biotherapiques Nosodes*. Volumes 1 & 2. Paris: Libraire le François.

Julian O A (1995). *Intestinal Nosodes of Bach-Paterson*. Translated by Kumar Mukerji R. New Delhi: B Jain Publishers.

Julian O A (1983). *Materia Medica der Nosoden*. Heidelberg: Haug.

Kayne L (2006). *Personal communication*.

Kennedy C O (1954). Further Notes on the Bowel Nosodes. *British Homeopathic Journal*; **44**: 100–103.

Kent J T (1926). *Lesser Writings and Precepts*. London: Homeopathic Publishing Co.

Khan M T (2007). *Personal communication*.

Laing R (1995). Using the bowel Nosodes. *British Homeopathic Journal*; **84**: 21–25.

Land S T (2008). 20 Years ago: British Homeopathic Journal, April 1988. *Homeopathy*; **97**: 108–110.

Lilley D (2007). The Chronic miasms. In: Owen D (ed.). *Principles and Practice of Homeopathy* (Chapter 17). London: Churchill Livingstone/Elsevier.

Malcolm R (2007). *Systems and Symbiosis. The Bowel Nosodes Reappraised*. London: Academic Unit Royal London Homeopathic Hospital.

Malcolm R (2012). Case report. *Simile*. Spring 2012.

Medical Research Council (1909). System of Bacteriology. *MRC*; **4**: 260.

Medina B, Girard I D, Jacotot E *et al* (2002). Effect of a preparation of Saccharomyces cerevisiae on microbial profiles and fermentation patterns in the large intestine of horses fed a high fibre or high starch diet. *J Anim Sci*; **80**: 2600–2609.

Moayyedi P *et al* (2017). Transplantation for C Difficile associated diarrhoea; a systemic review of randomised controlled trials. *Medical Journal Australia*; **207**(4) 166–172.

Morrison R (1993). *Desktop Guide to Keynotes and Confirmatory Symptoms*. Grass Valley, CA: Hahnemann Clinic Publishing.

Mount S J L (1973). On the Genesis, Nature and Control of Migraine. *British Homeopathic Journal*; **62**(3): 133–175.

Murphy R (1996). *Homeopathic Medical Repertory*. 2nd edn. Pagosa Springs CO: Hahnemann Academy of North America Press.

Murphy R (2000). *Homeopathic Remedy Guide*. Pagosa Springs CO: Hahnemann Academy of North America Press. (Originally published 1995 as *Lotus Materia Medica*.)

Neustaedter R (1988). Critique of the Bowel Nosodes. *British Homeopathic Journal*; **77**: 106–111.

Paramsothy *et al* (2018). Specific bacteria and metabolites associated with response to microbial transplant action in patients with ulcerative colitis. *Gastroenterology*; **156**(5): 1440–54.

Paterson E (1960). A Survey of the Nosodes. *British Homeopathic Journal*; **49**: 161–186.

Paterson J (1929). Psora in Children and the Use of Bach Nosodes. *British Homeopathic Journal*; **19**: 50–81.

Paterson J (1932). *Clinical notes and Observations on Twenty-two case from which a Diplococcus was isolated in stool culture*. Glasgow: Scottish Branch of Faculty of Homoeopathy. Nov 15th.

Paterson J (1933a). *A modern Conception of Homoeopathy*. London: Royal London Homoeopathic Hospital. Oct 12th.

Paterson J (1933b). Sycosis and Sycotic Co. *British Homeopathic Journal*; **23**: 160.

Paterson J (1936a). Technique in the Preparation of the Non-Lactose Fermenting Nosodes of the Bowel and the Clinical Indications for their use. *Proceedings of International Homoeopathic Congress, Glasgow*. pp 214–244.

Paterson J (1936b). The Potentised Drug and its Action on the Bowel Flora. *British Homeopathic Journal*; **26**: 163–188.

Paterson J (1937). Indications for the Use of the Intestinal Nosodes in Diseases of Children. *British Homeopathic Journal*; **27**: 344–352.

Paterson J (1949a). Morgan-Gaertner, the Bowel Nosode Complementary to Lycopodium. *British Homeopathic Journal*; **39**: 91–94.

Paterson J (1949b). The Role of the Bowel Flora in Chronic Disease. *British Homeopathic Journal*; **39**: 69–83.

Paterson J (1950). The Bowel Nosodes. Proceedings of the International Homoeopathic League, August 1949. *British Homeopathic Journal*; **40**(3): 153–162.

Paterson J (1953). Up to Date with Nosodes. Glasgow: Faculty of Homoeopathy (Scottish Branch); April 22nd.

Pedalino C M V (2006). Homeopathic Medicines in Potency Cords. *Cultura Homeopatica*; **16**: 18–21.

Rehman A (ed.) (1997). *Encyclopaedia of Remedy Relationships in Homeopathy*. Heidelberg: Karl Haug.

Rettiger L F, Cheplin H A (1921). *A Treatise on the Transformation of the Intestinal Flora with Special Reference to the Implantation of B acidophilus* New Haven, CT: Yale University Press.

Sankaran P (1984). *Indications and Uses of Bowel Nosodes*. Mumbai: Homeopathic Medical Publishers.

Saxton J, Gregory P (2005). *Textbook of Veterinary Homeopathy*. Beaconsfield, UK: Beaconsfield Publishers.

Saxton J (1994). Bowel Nosodes in Animals. *Proceedings of the AVHMA Congress, Orlando, FL*.

Saxton J (2005). Do we truly understand vaccine reactions and vaccinosis? *Homeopathy*; **94**: 200–201.

Saxton J (2006). *Miasms as Practical Tools*. Beaconsfield, UK: Beaconsfield Publishers.

Scholten J (1996). *Homeopathy and the Elements*. Utrecht, NL: Stichting Alonniss.

Schroyens F (ed.). (2004). *Synthesis: The Source Repertory, ed. 9.1.* London: Homeopathic Book Publishers.

Shaw G B (1937). *The Complete Plays.* London: Odhams Press Ltd.

Sherr J Y (2002). *Dynamic Materia Medica: Syphilis.* Malvern, UK: Dynamis Books.

Somper J D (1988). Some Cases in use of Bowel Nosodes. *British Homeopathic Journal*; 77: 82–80.

Somper J D (2002). *Personal communication.*

Swayne J (ed.) (2000). *International Dictionary of Homeopathy.* Edinburgh: Churchill Livingstone.

Tyler M L (1933). *Hahnemann's Concept of Chronic Disease as Caused by Parasitic Microorganisms.* London: John Bale & Danielson. Reprinted 2004 New Delhi: B Jain Publishers.

Treuherz F (1995). Bowel Nosode Keynotes. *Personal lecture material handout.*

Vermeulen F (2002). *Prisma: the Arcana of Materia Medica.* Haarlem, NL: Emryss bv Publishers.

Vermeulen F (2006). *Nosodes: a serial article part 1.* IAVH Newsletter; 3rd June.

Von Schreiber C I (2008). *Personal communication.*

Weeks N (c1940). *The Dr Edward Bach Remedies.* Talk given to the British Society of Dowsers. Wallingford UK Dr Edward Bach Centre. Available online at http://tinyurl.com/7tzdf8q

Wheeler C E (1924). A New Nosode. *British Homeopathic Journal*; 14: 164–189.

Yasgur J (1998). *Homeopathic Dictionary and Holistic Health Reference.* 4th edn. Greenville, PA: Van Hoy Publishers.

INDEX

Remedies included are those that are mentioned in the text. Remedies that are mentioned only in the associated remedy lists can be found in the appendix.